Behavioral Sleep Medicine

Lisa Medalie

Behavioral Sleep Medicine

A Practical Guide for Adult and Pediatric Providers

With Contributions by David Gozal
and Kathryn Hansen
Foreword by Hrayr Attarian

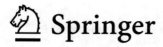 Springer

Lisa Medalie
Behavioral Sleep Medicine
DrLullaby
Chicago, IL, USA

ISBN 978-3-031-12576-8   ISBN 978-3-031-12574-4   (eBook)
https://doi.org/10.1007/978-3-031-12574-4

This Springer imprint is published by the registered company Springer Nature Switzerland AG
The registered company address is: Gewerbestrasse 11, 6330 Cham, Switzerland

This book is dedicated to the late Thomas Hobbins, M.D., who stirred my passion for the sleep field at the age of 17. It is also for my loving parents, Betty Slavin Medalie and George Robert Medalie, M.D., whose unstinting support and guidance paved the way for my career passion.

- L.M.

Foreword

"Doc, I have tried so many medications and nothing works." As a sleep physician, this is a complaint we hear far too often. Less than ideal sedative hypnotic efficacy is not only encountered in clinical practice, but also demonstrated in meta-analyses. The most recent publication on this shows modest improvement in sleep metrics when compared to placebo in almost all currently available prescription sleep medications [1]. As significant as the effectiveness problem is the safety issues with these drugs, which are, perhaps, more consequential. These include higher risk of dementia and mortality as well as falls particularly in older people [2].

To say that chronic insomnia, or the difficulty falling asleep and/or staying asleep for 3 months or more, is a prevalent disorder, is an understatement. Conservatively speaking, chronic insomnia affects 10% of the population, [3] it is the number one complaint in sleep clinics, [4] and sleep difficulties are second only to pain as presenting symptoms in primary care [5]. This common disorder also has a large impact on society. Chronic insomnia is expensive; in the USA, it has estimated to cost between $92.45 and $107.53 billion per year [6] in healthcare utilization. It is associated with poor quality of life to a degree comparable with chronic pain and diabetes [7]. Insomnia also increases the risk of cardiovascular and psychiatric comorbidities [8].

There is, however, an effective and safe treatment for chronic insomnia called Cognitive Behavioral Therapy for insomnia (CBT-I). It is a well-established modality delivered by providers with their own board certification and professional society, called Society of Behavioral Sleep Medicine (SBSM). In addition, CBT and related techniques can help a host of sleep conditions beyond chronic insomnia, including CPAP therapy adherence, nightmares, parasomnias, and circadian rhythm disorders. The reason that it remains far from ubiquitous is the lack of qualified practitioners. The University of Pennsylvania website lists 480 BSM specialists worldwide, most of whom are in the USA [9]. Even then, however, these practitioners are concentrated in few large urban areas with several states having no trained BSM specialists. Moreover, there is a lack of awareness among most healthcare providers about the existence and importance of the field of behavioral sleep medicine [10].

There are helpful apps and virtual offerings that are available and guide patients through self-directed programs; however, these are not always perceived as cost-effective by consumers [11] and most only address insomnia. One of these virtual offerings, DrLullaby™, includes access to a live, trained therapiss and hence can address other sleep issues as well. Another of its unique features is that it has resources for both adults and children experiencing sleep problems. The founder of this program, Lisa Medalie, PsyD, DBSM is a pioneer in this field as she is one of the few who are certified in both pediatric and adult BSM. She is also deeply passionate about expanding access to BSM not only to the USA but to the rest of the world through creative means such as telemedicine. This book is one large step towards that goal and, given her credentials Dr. Medalie is the best qualified person to write this extremely user friendly and instructive guide to BSM. The tome provides healthcare providers with well-researched behavioral sleep medicine techniques to address insomnia in all age groups, improve CPAP adherence, treat nightmares, and other parasomnias and advance circadian rhythms. Dr. Medalie has included in it easy to follow tips and detailed, step by step, recommendations for addressing this wide variety of sleep complaints. Other singular features are the quality, the abundance, and the practicality of the illustrations giving further credence to the age-old adage that a picture is worth a thousand words.

This practical guide is divided into nine chapters. The first chapter walks the reader through the process of performing CBT-I with helpful resources and diagrams. The second is dedicated to pediatric BSM. The third teaches the utility and the interpretation of actigraphy, an informative diagnostic tool that is often overlooked. Chapter 4 teaches CPAP adherence techniques, while 5 is about Imagery Rehearsal Therapy (IRT) for nightmares. The sixth chapter is on phase shifting therapy for delayed sleep phase disorder, the seventh is on night eating syndrome, the eighth on a variety of parasomnias, and the last is a list of BSM resources. Each section has at the end, a list of key articles on the individual topics for those who want to delve deeper into the particular knowledge area.

There are other BSM books available; however, there are many attributes that make Dr. Medalie's stand out of the crowd. In addition to the author's rare combination of clinical skills and competencies spanning all age groups, this volume is edited by two of the foremost authorities in sleep medicine: Dr. David Gozal, M.D., Ph.D. who needs no introduction, and Kathryn Hansen the executive director of the Society of Behavioral Sleep Medicine. Last but not least, the breadth of disorders covered here is unprecedented.

Having practiced sleep medicine in four different, academic, tertiary referral centrals for 23 years, I have often acutely felt the need for BSM services for my patients. I have been fortunate enough to have worked closely with several superbly skilled and compassionate individuals one of whom has been Dr. Medalie. Not all my colleagues, especially those in more resource limited settings, have been that lucky. I believe *Behavioral Sleep Medicine: A Practical Guide for Adult and Pediatric Providers* is a superlative and essential publication that will help remedy some of the shortage of BSM therapies. So that next time, a patient lists pharmacological agents they have tried and failed this handbook will give their healthcare provider the tools to administer novel, safe, and effective therapeutic modalities.

References

1. Zheng X, He Y, Yin F, Liu H, Li Y, Zheng Q, Li L. Pharmacological interventions for the treatment of insomnia: quantitative comparison of drug efficacy. Sleep Med. 2020;72:41-49. doi: https://doi.org/10.1016/j.sleep.2020.03.022. PMID: 32544795.

2. Choi JW, Lee J, Jung SJ, Shin A, Lee YJ. Use of Sedative-Hypnotics and Mortality: A Population-Based Retrospective Cohort Study. J Clin Sleep Med. 2018;14(10):1669-1677. doi: https://doi.org/10.5664/jcsm.7370. PMID: 30353805.

3. Morin CM, Drake CL, Harvey AG, Krystal AD, Manber R, Riemann D, Spiegelhalder K. Insomnia disorder. Nat Rev Dis Primers. 2015;1:15026. doi: https://doi.org/10.1038/nrdp.2015.26. PMID: 27189779.

4. Schutte-Rodin S, Broch L, Buysse D, Dorsey C, Sateia M. Clinical guideline for the evaluation and management of chronic insomnia in adults. J Clin Sleep Med. 2008;4(5):487-504. PMID: 18853708.

5. Culpepper L. Insomnia: a primary care perspective. J Clin Psychiatry. 2005;66 Suppl 9:14-7; quiz 42-3. PMID: 16336037.

6. Reynolds SA, Ebben MR. The Cost of Insomnia and the Benefit of Increased Access to Evidence-Based Treatment: Cognitive Behavioral Therapy for Insomnia. Sleep Med Clin. 2017;12(1):39-46. doi: https://doi.org/10.1016/j.jsmc.2016.10.011. PMID: 28159096.

7. Olfson M, Wall M, Liu SM, Morin CM, Blanco C. Insomnia and Impaired Quality of Life in the United States. J Clin Psychiatry. 2018;79(5):17m12020. doi: https://doi.org/10.4088/JCP.17m12020. PMID: 30256547.

8. Taylor DJ, Lichstein KL, Durrence HH. Insomnia as a health risk factor. Behav Sleep Med. 2003;1(4):227-47. doi: https://doi.org/10.1207/S15402010BSM0104_5. PMID: 15600216.

9. https://www.med.upenn.edu/cbti/provder_directory.html accessed 1/14/2022

10. Ulmer CS, Bosworth HB, Beckham JC, Germain A, Jeffreys AS, Edelman D, Macy S, Kirby A, Voils CI. Veterans Affairs Primary Care Provider Perceptions of Insomnia Treatment. J Clin Sleep Med. 2017;13(8):991-999. doi: https://doi.org/10.5664/jcsm.6702. PMID: 28728623

11. Bonin EM, Beecham J, Swift N, Raikundalia S, Brown JS. Psycho-educational CBT-Insomnia workshops in the community. A cost-effectiveness analysis alongside a randomised controlled trial. Behav Res Ther. 2014 Apr;55:40-7. doi: https://doi.org/10.1016/j.brat.2014.01.005.PMID: 24607500.

Hrayr Attarian
Feinberg School of Medicine
Northwestern University
Chicago, IL, USA

Introduction

The purpose of this workbook is to guide providers in their treatment of patients with behavioral sleep complaints. This work aims to provide structure to supervised hours for the Behavioral Sleep Medicine board examination. The Society for Behavioral Sleep Medicine offers our board examination. To sit for this board examination, trainees must complete 1,000 supervised hours.

Supervised hours are an essential part of learning to provide evidence-based treatment for complex Behavioral Sleep Medicine patients.

To identify a supervisor for your hours in Behavioral Sleep Medicine, it is first important to decide whether you have interest in working with adults, pediatrics, or both populations. Very few supervisors treat both populations. The Society for Behavioral Sleep Medicine is an excellent resource for identifying available supervisors. Dr. Medalie continues offers supervision and supervised hours to both adult and pediatric providers.

This workbook aims to support Behavioral Sleep Medicine trainees, undergoing supervised hours in preparation for their board examination. Those who recently took their board examination and are new to treating Behavioral Sleep Medicine patients will also find value in this workbook.

To optimize the benefits of this workbook, please use it in clinic with your patients. We intend for the "Clinic Talking Points" and modifiable "Patient Handouts," to be open with you while seeing patients. Dr. Medalie provides the talking points she has utilized for over 15 years in adult and pediatric clinics.

Dr. Medalie's talking points and handouts include her own professional style for delivering evidence-based behavioral strategies and are not meant to replace the importance of learning the methodologies directly from the original papers. The reading lists at the end of each strategy are offered to learn more about each technique. Once you have fully digested the research on each technique, you may find yourself modifying Dr. Medalie's clinic talking points and handouts to languages and styles that meet your own professional style. The purpose of this workbook is not to create a "cookie cutter" approach to Behavioral Sleep Medicine, but instead provide a launch-pad for new providers.

Acknowledgments

We'd like to acknowledge the **Society for Behavioral Sleep Medicine** for their constant dedication to supporting providers, disseminating resources, and developing accreditation processes which establish the gold-standard for training, assessment, and treatment.

The following individuals indirectly or directly supported the completion of this work:

Stori Stefanac

Sean Drummond, PhD

Carla Nappi, PhD

Daniel Lewin, PhD

Robert Thomas, MD

Babak Mokhlesi, MD

Hari Bandla, MD

Gina Richman, PhD

Andrew Zabel, PhD

Kate Kane, PhD

Kevin Adley, RPSGT, CCSH

Contents

Cognitive Behavioral Treatment for Insomnia

1

1.1 Visit 1: Intake and Sleep Hygiene

This section shows the process for the first visit in the CBT-I protocol. Our "Visit 1" typically entails a thorough assessment of the presenting complaints, sleep history, psychiatric and medical history, medication review and conceptualization of the diagnosis and plans for treatment. We also review tips for improving sleep hygiene during Visit 1, without describing any interventions that might bias our baseline data collection.

1.1.1 Provider Intake Form

This form is an example of a note taking form that a Behavioral Sleep Medicine specialist might use during a first visit with a referred patient. Note: *Additional data might be warranted for certain CPT codes—the content below only supports the data collection for case conceptualization of an insomnia patient (e.g., psychiatric diagnostic evaluation without medical services 90791 also warrants mental status evaluation).*

ADULT INSOMNIA INTAKE FORM	
Demographic	Patient Name: ***
	DOB: ***
	Age: ***
	Gender: ***
	Address: ***
	Phone: ***
	Email: ***
Sleep symptoms	
Current sleep symptoms	Brief description: ***
	Frequency: ***
	Onset: ***

© The Author(s), under exclusive license to Springer Nature Switzerland AG 2022
L. Medalie, *Behavioral Sleep Medicine*,
https://doi.org/10.1007/978-3-031-12574-4_1

ADULT INSOMNIA INTAKE FORM

Sleep schedule	Bedtime: ***
	Length of time to fall asleep: ***
	Number of awakenings: ***
	Duration of awakenings: ***
	Parent involvement with sleep: ***
	Waketime: ***
	Out of bed: ***
	Nap time/duration: ***
3 P's	Predisposing factors: ***
	Precipitating events: ***
	Perpetuating factors: ***
Sleep medication	Current medications (OTC or prescribed): ***
	Frequency of use: ***
	When started: ***
	Previous medications tried: ***
Sleep hygiene	Electronics (in bedroom, access during the night): ***
	White noise: ***
	Light: ***
	Caffeine: ***
	Alcohol: ***
	Marijuana: ***
	Nicotine: ***
	Partner co-sleeping: ***
Medically based sleep symptoms	Previous sleep study findings: ***
	Sleep apnea symptoms: ***
	Restless leg symptoms: ***
	Narcolepsy symptoms: ***
	Parasomnias: ***
Psychiatric	
Current mental health symptoms/diagnoses	***
Therapy - current therapy, hospitalization history, therapy history/ experience	***
Medication—current mood medications, history of medications	***
Medical	
Medical diagnoses/ physical symptoms	***
Current Medications - particular emphasis on medications contributing to insomnia or EDS	***
Impressions/plan	
Diagnosis	***
Treatment goals	***
Treatment plan/referrals	***

1.1.2   Intake Script

Current Sleep Symptoms
- Are you having trouble more with falling asleep, returning to sleep, or both?
- How many nights per week are you struggling?
- How long ago did this problem with sleep begin? What was going on in your life at that time?

Sleep Schedule
- Let's talk about your sleep schedule—what time do you close your eyes and try for sleep? Please give me a range—what is the earliest time and what is the latest time?
- How long will it take you to fall asleep after closing your eyes? Again, please provide a range—what is the shortest length of time it might take, and what is the longest?
- How many times will you wake during the night? What is the range there?
- How long are you awake if you add together those nighttime awakenings? What is the shortest length of time you are awake, and what is the longest you might be awake if you add together your nighttime awakenings?
  - If your patient reports "I do not return to sleep"—explain the difference between nighttime awakenings and early morning awakenings
    Nighttime awakenings occur when patients wake for a stretch of time during the night, but then at some point, they return to sleep.
    Early morning awakenings occur when patients wake at some point and then never return to sleep that day.
- For pediatric intakes: what is happening during the time your child is falling asleep or returning to sleep? Are you holding them, rocking them, feeding them, cuddling them, laying with them, etc? Are they in your bed or their bed? Any crying, screaming, or tantrums?
- What time will you wake for the final time in the morning?
- What is the range of time you might be awake before you get out of bed to start your day?
- How many days per week will you nap? How long are those naps?

3 P's
- Predisposing factors: Do you have any family history of insomnia? Early childhood symptoms of sleep disturbance? Any early childhood mood or behavior problems? Or early trauma exposure?
- Precipitating events: How many years ago did your insomnia start? What was going on at that time?
  - If your patient reports "I do not know"—let them know, it does not need to be a horrific problem or stressor, sometimes even schedule changes, illness or medication change can trigger such onset

Let's think back to that time, tell me more about what was going on in your life? Any changes, even if subtle? Let's really think this through as this data will be helpful in my preparation to help you.

- Perpetuating factors: While you are laying in bed trying for sleep, what type of thoughts might come up? After you have been laying there for a while, how might you feel emotionally? Is it more sad, angry, anxious, frustrated, etc? Are there any other factors that you can think of that might keep this problem going?

Sleep Medication
- What are you currently taking for sleep? When was this started? How many nights per week? Who prescribes this medication? What is the dosage?
- Prior to this medication, what else have you tried? What made you stop those medications?

Sleep Hygiene
- What are you typically doing during the hour before bedtime?
- What electronics are in your bedroom? What devices do you use between bedtime and waketime?
- Is there any noise that interferes with sleep? Have you tried white noise, or ear plugs?
- Is there any light that interferes with sleep? Have you tried an eye mask or blackout shades?
- How many caffeinated beverages might you have per day, or week? What is the latest you will have a caffeinated beverage?
- How many nights per week will you consume alcohol? How many drinks in a sitting? What time do you typically drink alcohol?
- Are you currently using marijuana? How much do you consume per day, or week? What time do you typically consume marijuana?
- Do you consume nicotine? Quantity? Timing?
- Do you have a bed partner? Does their sleep impact your sleep?

Psychiatric History
- Do you currently carry any mental health diagnosis? What are the current symptoms? Any depressive or anxiety symptoms currently?
- Are you currently in therapy? How often do you go? When were you last seen by a therapist (if not current)? How many therapists total?
- Have you ever had a psychiatric or substance related hospitalization? When was that? If depressive symptoms are endorsed—or any concerns about risk—ask, have things been so bad lately, that you've had any thoughts about ending your life? Query signs of intent or plan.
- Are you currently taking any medications to support mood? Which medications? Dosage? If not, any in the past?

Medical History
- Do you currently have any medical diagnoses? What are your current symptoms? Any pain? Reflux? Allergies? Irritable bowel? Hypertension?
- What is the current approach to treatment for such issues?

Medically-Based Sleep Symptoms
1. **Previous Sleep Studies**
   (a) Have you ever had a sleep study?
   (b) How many years ago was the study?
   (c) Has your weight changed since that time?
   - If more than 10% weight change, they might want to ask their sleep MD if a repeat study is appropriate; if it's been several years, they likewise might want to ask if a repeat study would be appropriate
   (d) Any diagnoses revealed from the study?
   (e) What treatment was suggested? Are you adherent?
   - **If sleep apnea**—do you know the Apnea Hypopnea Index (AHI)? Do you know if it was mild, moderate or severe?
     - **If pap**—how many nights per week are you wearing pap? How many nights per week are you wearing PAP? How many hours per night?
       For those patients not wearing PAP from bedtime to waketime— please see the chapter on PAP adherence and ask the specific questions to find out what the barriers to adherence are, so you can customize your CBT for PAP adherence treatment plan (i.e., motivation, claustrophobia, mood symptoms, equipment—mask, hose, machine, etc).
2. **Sleep Apnea Symptoms**
   (a) Do you snore? Is the snoring loud enough to be heard outside the bedroom? Is it frequent?
   (b) Do you wake up choking or gasping? Any pauses in breathing?
   (c) If bed partner, ask them to join the session and ask them these questions— most patients do not know if they are snoring or choking/gasping
   (d) Do you wake with a dry mouth?
   (e) Headache that goes away on it's own?
   (f) Frequent unintentional dozing during the day?
3. **Restless Leg Symptoms**
   (a) Any tingling or numbness in your legs while you are trying for sleep?
   (b) If I asked you to lay perfectly still in bed at night would you be able to do so?
   (c) Is this the reason you are struggling with sleep?
       If we got rid of this problem, would you still have insomnia?
4. **Narcolepsy Symptoms**
   (a) Sleep paralysis: Do you ever wake in the morning and feel like your mind is awake, but you can't move your body, almost like you are paralyzed?
   (b) Hypnagogic/Hypnopompic hallucinations: Do you ever see vivid or shadowy objects in the room while you are falling asleep or while you are waking up? Almost like parts of your dreams?
   (c) Cataplexy: Do you ever experience a strong emotion—like you are about to laugh really hard, and all of a sudden you lose muscle tone? Like your legs buckle?
   (d) Sleep attacks: Will you, out of nowhere, suddenly fall into deep sleep (i.e., eating, talking, etc)?

5. **Parasomnia Symptoms**
   (a) Any sleepwalking or odd behaviors during sleep?
   (b) If they reported a history of trauma previously:
      • Do you have nightmares 3 or more times per week? Has this happened
        for at least 3 months? Are they like horror movies in your dreams? Are
        you afraid to fall asleep or return to sleep? Frequent fear thoughts about
        these nightmares during the day?
   (c) Night terrors vs nightmares for kids:
      • What time of night do these events occur? Is their recall the next day?
        Can you calm down your child during the events? Do they recognize
        you? Can they engage in sensical speech (i.e., can they say something
        that makes sense)? [no replies and events in the first 3rd of the night are
        more indicative of night terrors]

6. **Diagnosis:**
   (a) From everything you have shared it sounds like you meet the criteria for
        Chronic Insomnia
   (b) We can make this diagnosis based on patient report of symptoms
   (c) Since you have symptoms 3 or more nights per week, for at least 3 months,
        and noted significant distress or impact on functioning, you meet our criteria
        for Chronic Insomnia
   (d) We understand your diagnosis based on the 3 P's we assessed:
      • Many times patients with insomnia have predisposing factors—for you,
        you noted _____. Just because predisposing factors or risk factors are
        present, does not mean that you will right away manifest symptoms.
      • It is typically not until the 2nd P, the precipitating event occurs, that
        patients experience their first bout of insomnia. For you, you noted ___
        as a significant change or stressor.
      • Just because the precipitating event occurred, does not explain why you
        still have symptoms today. This is where the perpetuating factors come
        in—you mentioned that you experience _____. We know that the mal-
        adaptive behaviors and patterns which emerge in the face of insomnia,
        which patients are often doing to deal with the insomnia, and/or result
        from night after night of sleep problems, can be the factors that keep the
        insomnia going.
      • While we can not do anything about your predisposing factors, as you
        were born with such risks, and we also can not stop you from having
        significant life stressors again in your life, we can help address the per-
        petuating factors and teach you the evidence-based strategies that are
        first-line for reducing your insomnia.

7. **Treatment Overview**
   (a) We will utilize a protocol called Cognitive Behavioral Treatment for Insomnia (CBT-I) to address your symptoms.
   (b) This is typically a 5–8 session protocol, but can be as many as 8–10 sessions when combined with sleep medication tapering (see Sect. 1.2.1).
   (c) CBT-I is kind of like physical therapy for your sleep—we will go through habit changes, and ways to improve control over thoughts and emotions, to more effectively see you succeed with sleep.
   (d) Research shows that CBT-I is actually the first-line treatment and gold standard for managing Chronic Insomnia. In fact, research shows that sleep medications should only be considered after someone does not respond to CBT-I, but 70–80% of patients do see results. The main reason people often end up on sleep medications first, is moreso an issue of insufficient access to CBT-I, as sleeping pills are not the first-line treatment recommended for Chronic Insomnia.
   (e) I expect you to feel skeptical about the likelihood of us being able to help— this is quite normal. I am not here to convince you that you should believe that we can fix your insomnia, but am hoping you are willing to at least try the protocol that does help most people with a similar issue.
   (f) While we go through this protocol, we will also assign changes to work on between sessions, and have you keep sleep logs throughout.
   (g) The sleep logs should be completed first thing in the morning.
   (h) We do not want you to look at the clock at all during the night to fill in your sleep logs. If there is a clock in your room, you can turn it around, or put something over it, as time thoughts are one of the most frequent types of thoughts that keep patients awake at night (e.g., what time is it, how much time has it been, how much time until morning, etc).
   (i) We understand that without looking at the clock, this might impact accuracy, and that is ok—we are mainly interested in your experience and your perception of your sleep. As well, as long as you are the one filling in your sleep logs each morning, we can measure change since we will compare your data to your data in each visit.
   (j) Also as a next step, I will review appropriate sleep hygiene changes for you to make between today and your next session (see Sect. 1.1.3).
   (k) We also want to be sure that you allow yourself to "turn your sleep over" to the protocol—i.e., try your best to robotically go through the motions of the changes, instead of continuing to "try to sleep". The only people out there "trying to sleep" are our insomnia patients. The irony of insomnia is the effort to sleep, is one of the main reasons you are continuing to struggle with sleep. If you can shift to letting go of your effort to sleep, that is at least half of the battle!

1.1.3   Sleep Hygiene Clinic Talking Points

- **Diet:**
  - Avoid heavy or spicy foods within 3 h of bedtime
  - You don't want to go to bed right after eating something heavy as your body will then go into "digestive mode" which would interfere with sleep continuity
  - You also don't want to go to bed hungry so a light snack before bed is reasonable
- **Exercise:**
  - People who exercise regularly sleep better
  - Minimize exercise within 3 h of bedtime
- **Electronics**
  - Blue light tells the brain to stop producing Melatonin
  - The content in devices is also too engaging
  - We suggest turning off devices 1 h before bedtime
  - Leave all devices charging outside of the bedroom
- **Light**
  - Consider use of an eye-mask or blackout shades
- **Pre-sleep ritual**
  - Repeating the same 3 step process nightly before bedtime
      1-hour of "me-time" to lower the somatic arousal system before trying for sleep
      Soft music, light reading, hot bath/shower
  - The hot bath/shower before bedtime can position your body temperature in the right place for sleep -when submerged in hot water, your body temperature rises, when you step out, there is a rapid drop in the core body temperature which is the ideal place for sleep
- **Room temperature**
  - People sleep best in cool temperature rooms—high 60's, low 70's is ideal for sleep
- **Noise**
  - Use a white noise machine from bedtime to waketime
  - In-room units are ideal since we want the bedtime charging out of the bedroom
  - You can use a white noise app for traveling
  - We suggest a constant loud sound (e.g., white, pink, brown noise, etc.), as opposed to fluctuating background sounds (e.g., beach, rainforest, etc.), as the mind can habituate to a constant sound, but our mind follows the sound fluctuations of sound deviations such as a random bird chirp, which then interferes with sleep
- **Caffeine/alcohol/nicotine/marijuana**
  - We suggest minimizing caffeine 6–10 h before bedtime; ideally after noon
      Caffeine half-life varies from one person to the next
  - Minimize use of "night caps"—while this might initially decrease sleep onset time, it can be habit-forming, and alcohol generally has a negative impact on sleep architecture, increases sleep apnea/RLS (if present), and leaves you waking feeling more groggy
  - Nicotine is a stimulant and should be avoided before bedtime and during the night

– We still do not have consistent well-designed RCT's supporting the use of marijuana for sleep

Use of CBT-I continues to be the first-line recommendation for improving insomnia

The Figs. 1.1, 1.2, 1.3, 1.4, 1.5, 1.6, 1.7, 1.8, 1.9, 1.10 and 1.11**, patient handouts, clinic talking points, and diagnostic criteria are shown below to help with the understanding and working with Cognitive Behavioral Treatment for Insomnia (CBT-I).**

1.1.4   Sleep Hygiene Patient Handout

This is a handout Dr. Medalie shares with insomnia patients at the culmination of their first CBT-I session to remind them of changes to make before their 2nd visit.

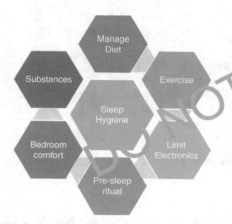

Diet: Avoid heavy meals within 3 hours of bedtime

Exercise: Regular exercise supports optimal sleep - minimize exercise within 3 hours of bedtime

Electronics: Turn off devices 1 hour before bedtime - leave them off

Pre-sleep ritual: Hot bath/shower, soft music, light reading before bedtime

Bedroom comfort: White noise machine, cool temperature, black-out shades

Substances: Minimize "night caps", limit nicotine before bedtime/during sleep window, stop caffeine 6-10 hours before bedtime

1.1.5   Chronic Insomnia Diagnostic Criteria

Chronic Insomnia Disorder

ICD-9-CM code: 307.42   ICD-10-CM code: F51.01

Diagnostic Criteria
Criteria A–E must be met
A. The patient reports, or the patient's parent or caregiver observes, one or more of the following:
   a. Difficulty initiating sleep.
   b. Difficulty maintaining sleep.
   c. Waking up earlier than desired.
   d. Resistance to going to bed on an appropriate schedule.
   e. Difficulty sleeping without parent or caregiver intervention.

B. The patient reports, of the patient's parent or caregiver observes, one or more of the following related to the nighttime sleep difficulty:
  a. Fatigue/malaise.
  b. Attention, concentration, or memory impairment.
  c. Impaired social, family, vocational, or academic performance.
  d. Mood disturbance irritability.
  e. Daytime sleepiness.
  f. Behavioral problems (e.g., hyperactivity, impulsivity, aggression).
  g. Reduced motivation/energy initiative.
  h. Proneness for errors/accidents.
  i. Concerns about or dissatisfaction with sleep.
C. The reported sleep/wake complaints cannot be explained purely by inadequate opportunity (i.e., enough time is allotted for sleep) or inadequate circumstances (i.e., the environment is safe, dark, quiet, and comfortable) for sleep.
D. The sleep disturbance and associated daytime symptoms occur at least three times per week.
E. The sleep disturbance and associated daytime symptoms have been present for less than 3 months
F. The sleep/wake difficulty is not better explained by another sleep disorder.

1.1.6   Short-Term Insomnia Diagnostic Criteria

Short-Term Insomnia Disorder

ICD-9-CM code: 307.41   ICD-10-CM code: F51.02

Alternate Names
Acute insomnia, adjustment insomnia.

Diagnostic Criteria
Criteria A–E must be met
A. The patient reports, or the patient's parent or caregiver observes, one or more of the following:
  a. Difficulty initiating sleep.
  b. Difficulty maintaining sleep.
  c. Waking up earlier than desired.
  d. Resistance to going to bed on an appropriate schedule.
  e. Difficulty sleeping without parent or caregiver intervention.

B. The patient reports, of the patient's parent or caregiver observes, one or more of the following related to the nighttime sleep difficulty:
   a. Fatigue/malaise.
   b. Attention, concentration, or memory impairment.
   c. Impaired social, family, vocational, or academic performance.
   d. Mood disturbance irritability.
   e. Daytime sleepiness.
   f. Behavioral problems (e.g., hyperactivity, impulsivity, aggression).
   g. Reduced motivation/energy initiative.
   h. Proneness for errors/accidents.
   i. Concerns about or dissatisfaction with sleep.
C. The reported sleep/wake complaints cannot be explained purely by inadequate opportunity (i.e., enough time is allotted for sleep) or inadequate circumstances (i.e., the environment is safe, dark, quiet, and comfortable) for sleep.
D. The sleep disturbance and associated daytime symptoms occur at least three times per week.
E. The sleep disturbance and associated daytime symptoms have been present for at least 3 months.
F. The sleep/wake difficulty is not better explained by another sleep disorder.

1.1.7   Other Insomnia Disorder Diagnostic Criteria

Other Insomnia Disorder

ICD-9-CM code: 307.49   ICD-10-CM code: F51.09

Diagnostic Criteria
This diagnosis is reserved for individuals who complain of difficulty initiating and maintaining sleep and yet do not meet the full criteria for either chronic insomnia disorder or short-term insomnia disorder. In some cases, this diagnosis may be assigned on a provisional basis when more information is needed to establish a diagnosis of chronic insomnia disorder or short-term insomnia disorder. It is expected that this diagnosis will be used sparingly, given its non-specific nature.

1.1.8   Cognitive Behavioral Treatment for Insomnia Sleep Log

Patient should keep sleep logs throughout the full course of Cognitive Behavioral Treatment for Insomnia

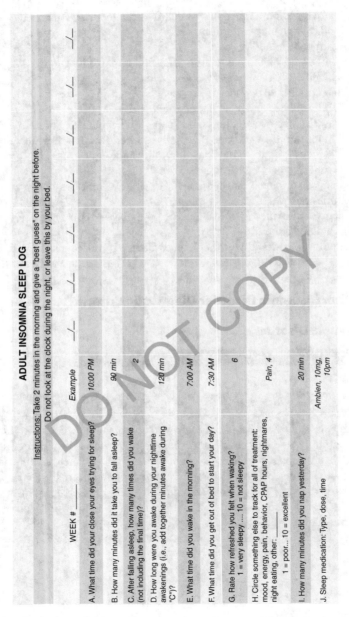

Fig. 1.1 This is a sleep log example Dr. Medalie used in clinic with insomnia patients to track their subjective experience of their sleep during CBT-I. Printing and use of this handout is not permitted unless directly approved by Dr. Medalie. If interested in accumulating BSM hours or referring patients, Dr. Medalie might be able to help—https://drlullaby.com/

1.1.9   Weekly Questionnaire for Cognitive Behavioral Treatment for Insomnia Sessions

Insomnia Severity Index

The Insomnia Severity Index has seven questions. The seven answers are added up to get a total score. when you have your total score. Look at the 'Guidelines for Scoring/Interpretation' below to see where your sleep difficulty fits.

For each question, please CIRCLE the number that best describes your answer.

Please rate the CURRENT (i.e. LAST 2 WEEKS) SEVERITY of your insomnia problem(s).

Insomnia Problem	None	Mild	Moderate	Severe	Very Severe
1. Difficulty falling asleep	0	1	2	3	4
2. Difficulty staying asleep	0	1	2	3	4
3. Problems waking up too early	0	1	2	3	4

4. How SATISFIED/DISSATISFIED are you with your CURRENT sleep pattern?

Very satisfied	Satisfied	Moderately Satisfied	Dissatisfied	Very dissatisfied
0	1	2	3	4

5. How NOTICEABLE to others do you think your sleep problem is in terms of impairing the quality of your life?

Not at all Noticeable	A little	Somewhat	Much	Very Much Noticeable
0	1	2	3	4

6. How WORRIED/DISTRESSED are you about your current sleep problem?

Not at all Worried	A little	Somewhat	Much	Very Much Worried
0	1	2	3	4

7. To what extent do you consider your sleep problem to INTERFERE with your daily functions (e.g. daytime fatigue, mood, ability to function at work/daily chores, concentration, memory, mood, etc.) CURRENTLY?

Not at all Interfering	A little	Somewhat	Much	Very Much Interfering
0	1	2	3	4

Guidelines for Scoring/Interpretation:

Add the scores for all seven items (questions 1 + 2 + 3 + 4 + 5 + 6 + 7) = _____ your total score

Total score categories:

0-7 = No clinically significant insomnia

8-14 = Subthreshold insomnia

15-21 = Clinical insonia (moderate level)

22-28 = Clinical insomnia (severe)

Fig. 1.2 This is a frequently used index for the assessment of distress response and functional impact of insomnia

1.1.10 Sleep Hygiene Reading List

Albakri U., Arnedt JT, Bertisch SM et al. (2021). Sleep health promotion interventions and their effectiveness: An umbrella review. *Int J Environ Res Public Health, May 21; 18* (11): 5533.

Chung, K.-F., Lee, C.-T., Yeung, W.-F., et al. (2018). Sleep hygiene education as a treatment of insomnia: A systematic review and meta-analysis. *Family Practice, 35*(4), 365–375.

Espie CA. (2021). The '5 principles' of good sleep health. *J Sleep Res, Oct 21:* e13502.

Edinger JD, Arnedt JT, Bertisch SM, et al. (2021). Behavioral and psychological treatments for chronic insomnia disorder in adults: an American Academy of Sleep Medicine clinical practice guideline. *J Clin Sleep Med, Feb 1; 17*(2): 255–262.

Hale D. & Marshall K. (2019). Sleep and Sleep Hygiene. *Home Healthc Now, Jul/ Aug;37*(4):227.

Hauri P. & Linde SM. (1996). *No more sleepless nights.* New York: Wiley.

Riemann D. (2018). Sleep hygiene, insomnia and mental health. *J Sleep Res, Feb;27*(1):3.

Stepanski, E. J., & Wyatt, J. K. (2003). Use of sleep hygiene in the treatment of insomnia. *Sleep Medicine Reviews, 7*(3), 215–225

Takano Y., Iwano S., Aoki S., et al. (2021). A systematic review of the effect of sleep interventions on presenteeism. *Biopsychosoci Med, 17; 15*(1): 21.

Zagaria A, Ballesio A., Ballesio A., et al. (2021). Psychometric properties of the sleep hygiene index in a large Italian community sample. *Sleep Med, Aug 84*: 362–367.

Zhang J, Xu Z, Zhao K, et al. (2018). Sleep Habits, Sleep Problems, Sleep Hygiene, and Their Associations With Mental Health Problems Among Adolescents. *J Am Psychiatr Nurses Assoc, May/Jun;24*(3):223–234.

1.2   Visit 1 Add-on (As Needed): Sleep Medication Taper

This section reviews how to talk to your patient about the sleep medication taper process and address common barriers to buy-in. Behavioral Sleep Medicine specialists might be trained to deliver CBT-I side-by-side with a gradual prescription sleep medication taper.

1.2.1   Medication Taper Clinic Talking Points

- It looks like you are taking ___ for sleep, what is your plan regarding medication?
- Are you interested in staying on this medication or tapering off this medication alongside CBT-I? Have you talked about this with your doctor?
- If you would like to gradually taper off medication alongside CBT-I, we first ask that you talk to your prescribing physician and make sure they approve of this plan—we are happy to provide details about a possible plan that can be utilized alongside our CBT-I program
- It is essential to never cold turkey stop a medication that you have been taking nightly
- Instead, Charles Morin, PhD has published on the best approach for tapering off sleep medications, which includes decreasing by 25% every 2 weeks, until you are down to the final quarter, then going to every-other-night on the final quarter, every 3rd night, then 1/week and then just leave the bottle in your medication cabinet and take the quarter as needed
- This is not something we would start until you get approval from your prescribing doctor—most patients completing a taper alongside CBT-I will start the first taper step at the time of "Visit #2"
- This full process typically takes 8–10 weeks and is best completed alongside CBT-I

Those taking multiple medications:
- Given that you are taking multiple medications, you will also need to talk to your prescribing physician about which to taper first
- Some patients will decrease all medications by 25% every 2 weeks, instead of going one after the other—please confirm with your prescribing physician which approach makes the most sense given where you are
- It is also important to make sure you are optimally managing co-morbid symptoms while we embark on this process—if for example, mood, pain, IBS, etc. is not optimally controlled, this taper process could be more challenging

- We will work on this slowly and together and most patients end up either tapering completely off their sleep aids, or at least getting to a significantly lower dose

If appropriate:
- Given that z-class drugs and anxiolytics are not recommended in patients over the age of 65 years old, due to increased risk for falls and cognitive effects, this is something we would need to do soon/should have done previously, anyways
- These medications are not intended or approved as long-term nightly used agents; therefore, it is great that you have decided to start this plan
- Given the habit-forming nature of these medications, and that CBT-I is the first line (it's recommended that CBT-I is tried before starting medications), it makes sense that we work on this taper schedule

1.2.2　Sleep Medication Taper Patient Handout

Medication Taper Plan	Ask your prescribing physician for approval before our next visit
	Decrease by 25% every 2 weeks until down the final quarter; then go to every other night on the final quarter, every 3 nights, 1/week and then take as needed
	We never want you to stop, cold-turkey, any sleep aid that you have used nightly
	Decide with your prescribing doctor whether you will taper one medication at a time (or reduce all by 25% every 2 weeks); and which to start with
	Common reasons for tapering: side effects, dependency and tolerance risks, many sleeping pills are not indicated after the age of 65 years, many are not intended for nightly or long-term use

Fig. 1.3 This is Dr. Medalie's example of a follow-up template used in clinic for pediatric follow-up visits

1.2.3   Sleep Medication Taper Reading List

Allary A, Proulx-Tremblay V, Bélanger C, et al. (2020). Psychological predictors of benzodiazepine discontinuation among older adults: Results from the PASSE 60. *Addict Behav. Mar;102*:106195.

Baillargeon L., Landreville P., Verreault R., et al. (2003). Discontinuation of benzodiazepines among older insomniac adults treated with cognitive behavioural therapy combined with gradual tapering: a randomized trial. *CMAJ, Nov 11:169*(10): 1015–20.

Belleville G., Guay C., Guay B. et al. (2007). Hypnotic taper with or without self-help treatment of insomnia: a randomized clinical trail. *J Consult Clin Psychol, Apr: 75*(2): 325–35.

Belleville G & Morin CM. (2008). Hypnotic discontinuation in chronic insomnia: impact of psychological distress, readiness to change, and self-efficacy. *Health Psychol. Mar;27*(2):239–48.

Beaulieu-Bonneau S., Ivers H., Guay B., et al. (2017). Long-term maintenance of therapeutic gains associated with cognitive behavioral therapy for insomnia delivered alone or combined with Zolpidem. *Sleep, Mar 1: 40*(3).

Belleville G. & Morin CM. (2008). Hypnotic discontinuation in chronic insomnia: impact of psychological distress, readiness to change, and self-efficacy. *Health Psychol. Mar 27*(2): 239–48.

Belanger L., Morin CM, Bastien C. et al. (2005). Self-efficacy and compliance with benzodiazepine taper in older adults with chronic insomnia. *Health Psychol, May: 24*(3): 281–7.

Gulyani, S., Salas, R. E., & Gamaldo, C. E. (2012). Sleep medicine pharmacotherapeutics overview. *Chest, 142*(6), 1659–1668.

Hood HK, Rogojanski J, & Moss TG. (2014). Cognitive-behavioral therapy for chronic insomnia. *Curr Treat Options Neurol., Dec;16*(12):321.

Hintze JP & Edinger JD. (2020). Hypnotic discontinuation in chronic insomnia. *Sleep Med Clin, Jun;15*(2):147–154.

Morin CM, Bastien C, Guay B et al. (2004). Randomized clinical trial of supervised tapering and cognitive behavior therapy to facilitate benzodiazepine discontinuation in older adults with chronic insomnia. *Am J Psychiatry, 161*(2); 332–42.

Morin CM, Belanger L., Bastien C., et al. (2005). Long-term outcome after discontinuation of benzodiazepines for insomnia: a survival analysis of relapse. *Behav Res Ther. Jan: 43*(1): 1–14.

Reeve E, Ong M, Wu A, et al. (2017). A systematic review of interventions to deprescribe benzodiazepines and other hypnotics among older people. *Eur J Clin Pharmacol. Aug;73*(8):927–935.

Riemann, D., & Perlis, M. L. (2009). The treatments of chronic insomnia: A review of benzodiazepine receptor agonists and psychological and behavioral therapies. Sleep Medicine Reviews, 13(3), 205–214.

Schroeck, J. L., Ford, J., Conway, E. L., et al. (2016). Review of safety and efficacy of sleep medicines in older adults. Clinical Therapeutics, 38(11), 2340–2372.

Wilson, S., Nutt, D., Alford, C., et al. (2010). British Association for Psychopharmacology consensus statement on evidence-based treatment of insomnia, parasomnias and circadian rhythm disorders. Journal of Psychopharmacology, 24(11), 1577–1601.

Wright A, Diebold J, Otal J, et al. (2015). The effect of Melatonin on benzodiazepine discontinuation and sleep quality in adults attempting to discontinue benzodiazepines: A systematic review and meta-analysis. *Drugs Aging. Dec;32*(12):1009–18.

1.3   Visit 2: Stimulus Control and Sleep Restriction

This section starts with an example of a form that can be used for taking follow-up visit notes. It then reviews the details of what to say to explain and implement stimulus control and sleep restriction.

1.3.1   Behavioral Sleep Medicine Follow-up Form

Use for all Behavioral Sleep Medicine follow-up visits

PROVIDER FOLLOW-UP FORM	
Demographic	Patient Name: *** DOB: *** Age: *** Gender: *** Address: *** Phone: *** Email: ***
Data	
Sleep log averages	Average total sleep time: *** Average time until asleep: *** Average time awake: *** Average sleep efficiency: ***
Treatment stage	
Previous strategies assigned/ comments on implementation	***
Updates/plan	
Upcoming strategies assigned	***
Updated goal	***
Plan discussed for addressing barriers/new referrals	***
COPY OF SLEEP LOG/ACTOGRAM	

Printing and use of this handout is not permitted unless directly approved by Dr. Medalie. If interested in accumulating BSM hours or referring patients, Dr. Medalie might be able to help—https://drlullaby.com/

1.3.2 Stimulus Control Clinic Talking Points

- Stay out of the bed from wake time until bedtime.
- Set up a "reading spot" in the bedroom, but no reading on the bed.
- Find the right reading material to put in the reading spot—interesting enough, but not a "page turner".
- After getting into bed at bedtime, if it feels like it has been 15–20 min (do not look at the clock, but if it feels like a bunch of time has passed), or as soon as you notice your mind racing, feelings frustrated, anxious or bothered, get out of bed and go to the reading spot. We want you to read for only 5–10 min (2–3 pages) max. The point of getting out of bed and reading is to get your mind off whatever you were thinking about in bed.
- After 5–10 min of reading, get back into bed.
- If again it feels like 15–20 min, or again you feel stressed or bothered, go back to the reading spot—keep repeating as needed.
- Repeat the same steps during nighttime awakenings or early morning awakenings.

1.3.3 Stimulus Control Patient Handout

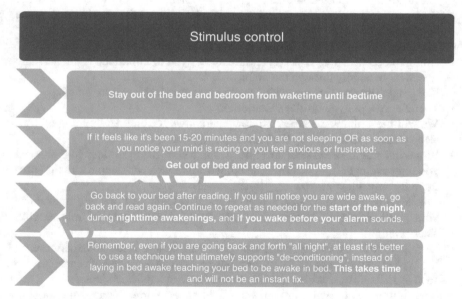

Fig. 1.4 This is Dr. Medalie's example of what she sends home with patients to remind them of changes related to stimulus control. Printing and use of this handout is not permitted unless directly approved by Dr. Medalie. If interested in accumulating BSM hours or referring patients, Dr. Medalie might be able to help—https://drlullaby.com/

1.3.4 Stimulus Control Reading List

Bootzin, R. R., Epstein D., Wood J. M., Stimulus control instructions. In Hauri, P. J. (1991). Case studies in insomnia. (pp.19–28). Springer.

Bootzin, R. R., & Perlis, M. L. (1992). Nonpharmacologic treatments of insomnia. Journal of Clinical Psychiatry, 53 Suppl, 37–41.

Brewster GS, Riegel B, Gehrman PR. Insomnia in the Older Adult. Sleep Med Clin. 2018 Mar;13(1):13–19.

Epstein, D. R., Sidani, S., Bootzin, R. R., & Belyea, M. J. (2012). Dismantling multicomponent behavioral treatment for insomnia in older adults: A randomized controlled trial. Sleep, 35(6), 797–805.

Morin CM, Hauri PJ, Espie CA, Spielman AJ, Buysse DJ, Bootzin RR. Nonpharmacologic treatment of chronic insomnia. An American Academy of Sleep Medicine review. Sleep. 1999 Dec 15;22(8):1134–56.

1.3.5 Sleep Restriction Clinic Talking Points

- Today we will also start you on something called "sleep restriction" which utilizes a concept of homeostatic sleep pressure, which is your body's urge for sleep.
- When you first wake in the morning, your relative drive for sleep is zero, since you just slept.
- The longer time you spend awake, the higher your sleep pressure builds.
- Going to bed with a high sleep pressure allows you to fall asleep faster and stay asleep more solidly through the night.
- The longer time you spend awake, the higher your sleep pressure builds.
- Therefore we put you on sleep restriction.
- We will prescribe you a sleep window that allows for optimal building of your sleep pressure to decrease your insomnia symptoms.
- While this might sound counterintuitive, since your baseline sleep logs showed you only averaged ____ hours of sleep, we will start your sleep restriction program by only allowing you ____ hours in bed.
- This level of sleep restriction is only temporary. Each visit, we will re-evaluate your sleep efficiency. If there is a nice boost, we will add 20 min to your sleep window.
- During your first week of sleep restriction, you should expect to experience all the typical experiences of sleep loss, but perhaps in a more noticeable way—such as irritability, trouble focusing, low energy, and appetite changes.
- Even if you do not typically nap, you might have an urge to nap while on your first week of sleep restriction. If this happens, this is sleep restriction working. Your sleep pressure is building, which is what we are trying for, but DO NOT NAP!
- We encourage complete nap avoidance throughout CBT-I—and ideally ongoing, given that people with insomnia are at risk for relapse of insomnia symptoms if they nap.

- We also encourage you to set an alarm, even if you feel you "don't need one". This will help to anchor your waketime and keep your schedule consistent.
- Sleep restriction is very hard to adhere to, so please do your best to stay motivated, and remember, you may initially feel worse, before you feel better.
- If/since we will not see you in 1 week, please feel free to add 20 min to your sleep window for your 2nd week. You can either go to bed 20 min earlier or sleep in 20 min later, depending on how your numbers look (i.e., you would not add 20 min to your bedtime if you had sleep onset troubles, and you would not add 20 min to your waketime if you had early morning awakenings). If you have seizures, history of mania, are a long-haul truck driver, sleep restriction is contraindicated.
- Remember you are allowed to stop if you need to!

1.3.6   Sleep Restriction Patient Handout

Sleep Restriction Plan

Sleep
schedule

Week 1: Bedtime _____ - Waketime _____
Week 2: Bedtime _____ - Waketime _____

> **Total nap avoidance** – dozing off or taking naps will decrease your sleep pressure which will make the results from sleep restriction less powerful

> **Morning alarm** - get immediately out of bed at your scheduled waketime. If you do not keep a consistent bedtime and waketime, this will also take away from the impact of sleep restriction.

Fig. 1.5 Dr. Medalie uses this handout to remind patients the changes related to sleep restriction. Printing and use of this handout is not permitted unless directly approved by Dr. Medalie. If interested in accumulating BSM hours or referring patients, Dr. Medalie might be able to help—https://drlullaby.com/

1.3.7   Sleep Restriction Reading List

Cheng P, Kalmbach D, Fellman-Couture C, et al. (2020). Risk of excessive sleepiness in sleep restriction therapy and cognitive behavioral therapy for insomnia: a randomized controlled trial. *J Clin Sleep Med. Feb 15;16*(2):193–198.

Kyle, S. D., Aquino, M. R. J., Miller, C. B., et al. (2015). Towards standardization and improved understanding of sleep restriction therapy for insomnia disorder: A systematic examination of CBT-I trial content. *Sleep Medicine Reviews, 23, 83–88.*

Lichstein, K. L., Thomas, S. J., & McCurry, S. M. (2011). *Sleep compression. In Behavioral Treatments for Sleep Disorders* (pp. 55–59). Elsevier.

Maurer L.F., Espie C.A., & Kyle S.D (2018). How does sleep restriction therapy for insomnia work? A systematic review of mechanistic evidence and the introduction of the Triple-R model. *Sleep Med Rev.*;42:127–138.

Maurer LF, Espie CA, Omlin X, et al. (2021). The effect of sleep restriction therapy for insomnia on sleep pressure and arousal: a randomised controlled mechanistic trial. *Sleep, Aug 31*:zsab223.

Maurer LF, Schneider J, Miller CB, et al. (2021). The clinical effects of sleep restriction therapy for insomnia: A meta-analysis of randomised controlled trials. *Sleep Med Rev. Aug;*58:101493

Miller CB, Espie CA, Epstein DR, et al. (2014). The evidence base of sleep restriction therapy for treating insomnia disorder. *Sleep Med Rev. Oct;18*(5):415–24.

Morin CM, Hauri PJ, Espie CA, et al. (1999). Nonpharmacologic treatment of chronic insomnia. An American Academy of Sleep Medicine review. *Sleep, Dec 15;22*(8):1134–56.

Spielman A.J, Saskin P. & Thorpy M.J., (1987). Treatment of chronic insomnia by restriction of time in bed. *Sleep;10*(1):45–56.

Whittall H, Pillion M, & Gradisar M. (2018). Daytime sleepiness, driving performance, reaction time and inhibitory control during sleep restriction therapy for Chronic Insomnia Disorder. *Sleep Med. May;45*:44–48.

1.4   Visit 3: Relaxation Strategies

This section outlines what to say to teach relaxation strategies to patients with insomnia. Diaphragmatic breathing, positive imagery and progressive muscle relaxation are reviewed.

1.4.1   Relaxation Strategies Clinic Talking Points

- Today we will review three main strategies to help lower your somatic arousal system and support transition into and back to sleep
  1. Diaphragmatic breathing
  2. Positive Imagery
  3. Progressive Muscle Relaxation
- For the first, sit back in your chair, close your eyes and put your hands on your belly—take a slow deep breath in through your nose and out through your

mouth—good. It should take you 3–4 s to slowly pull the air in, hold it for 1–2 s, and 3–4 s to slowly push the air out through your mouth. Picture the words "breathing in" while you inhale and "breathing out" while you exhale
- We want you to do 10 slow deep breaths to transition into sleep at the start of the night then again use 10 slow deep breaths to return to sleep during nighttime awakenings
- For the next, pick a place you have been to that makes you feel calm and relaxed—imagine it in full detail—what do you see, hear, taste and smell. Imagine a beginning, middle and end to that scene. While you are doing this, your mind will wander, and when it does, just imagine the thought floating off into a cloud, then gently bring yourself back to the calming scene
- For the last technique, you will go through each of the muscle groups in your body—and tense for 7 s, then relax for 7 s. Let's try it. Life your legs up and point your toes towards yourself, do you feel your calf muscles tightening up? Good, hold it for a bit longer, and now relax. Notice that difference between muscle tension and muscle relaxation—how nice it feels that those calf muscles are completely relaxed?
- Now imagine—if your muscles are all tensed up, your mind is racing, and your breathing is fast, it's not so easy to sleep!
- We want you to experiment with different techniques and find out which works best for you- use a strategy for transition into and back to sleep—these are great for prevention/use on a nightly basis
- Consider use of an MP3 player or Ipod for use of audio versions of these techniques (to keep your cell phone out of the bedroom)

1.4.2   Relaxation Strategies Patient Handout

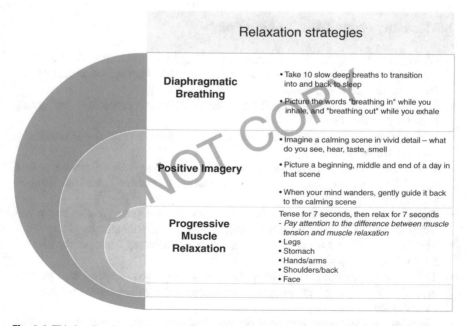

Fig. 1.6 This handout is what Dr. Medalie uses to remind patients how to try relaxation strategies in support of insomnia symptom reduction. Printing and use of this handout is not permitted unless directly approved by Dr. Medalie. If interested in accumulating BSM hours or referring patients, Dr. Medalie might be able to help—https://drlullaby.com/

1.4.3 Relaxation Strategies Reading List

Freedman R & Papsdorf JD (1976). Biofeedback and progressive relaxation treat-
    ment of sleep-onset insomnia: a controlled, all-night investigation. *Biofeedback
    Self Regul. Sep;1*(3):253–71.
Lehrer , P. M., Woolfolk, R. L., & Sime, W. E. (2007). *Principles and Practice of
    Stress Management (Third Edition)*. Guilford Press.
Means, M. K., Lichstein, K. L., Epperson, M. T., et al. (2000). Relaxation therapy
    for insomnia: Nighttime and daytime effects. *Behaviour Research and Therapy,
    38*(7), 665–678.
Meltzer, L.J., McLaughlin, & Crabtree, V. (2015). *Pediatric sleep problems: A clini-
    cian's guide to behavioral interventions*. American Psychological Association.
Nicassio PM, Boylan MB & McCabe TG (1982). Progressive relaxation, EMG bio-
    feedback and biofeedback placebo in the treatment of sleep-onset insomnia. *Br J
    Med Psychol. Jun;55*(Pt 2):159–66.
Ziv N, Rotem T, Arnon Z, et al. (2008). The effect of music relaxation versus pro-
    gressive muscular relaxation on insomnia in older people and their relationship
    to personality traits. *J Music Ther. Fall;45*(3):360–80.

1.5   Visit 4: Worry-time

We discuss the ways that Behavioral Sleep Medicine specialists might teach Worry-
time in this section.

1.5.1 Worry-time Clinic Talking Points

- We are now getting into the "C" part of the Cognitive Behavioral Treatment for
  Insomnia (CBT-I) sessions—we are going to start working on cognition, or
  thoughts, that keep you awake
- Many people with insomnia tend to think about worries or problems while laying
  in bed trying for sleep
- With our busy lives, we typically do not allow set time to process our worries or
  face our current problems
- Then when it's just you and your brain at night, and there is no cell phone, people
  or tasks to distract you, all of your problems or worries come bubbling to
  the surface
- The goal of worry-time is to schedule a time to face your worries and problems—get all of it out of your head well in advance of your sleep window
- We want you to sort through your worries or problems to decrease the content
  available to keep you awake
- This is different from a checklist of tasks as we want you to spend time coming
  up with solutions or plans for how to solve topics that might come up while you
  try for sleep
- We want you spend no less than 30 min, but more than 10 min on this daily
  exercise

- In the first column, make a list of all the worries or problems that might come up that night while you try for sleep—you know your brain and the types of worries or problems you think about or dwell on
- The second column is where you list 2–3 ways to either solve or cope with each one of these worries or problems
- Then the third column is after you've weighed the pros and cons for each of these potential solutions or coping strategies, and decided on an "action plan"—here is what I will do, when I will do it, and how I will do it
- Once you have an action plan for each worry or problem that might come up that night, you are done for the day
- If a worry or a problem comes up outside of your scheduled time, jot it down on an index card and put it aside with this notebook/papers/laptop—tell yourself, this it not the time for worry
- If a problem thought comes up while you are trying for sleep, use stimulus control or relaxation strategies
- It is important to compartmentalize when you allow yourself to worry and when you do not allow for worry focus
- This is meant to be a daily exercise, even if there is not much to put down on a particular day—and can be very helpful for our patients with insomnia

1.5.2 Worry-time Patient Handout

Worry-time Patient Handout		
Problem Solving Time	**Reminders:** - At least 3 hours before bedtime - Can use notebook, laptop, or voice recorder instead - 10-30 min daily exercise - Jot down new worries on an index card and save them for later if they come up outside of this time - If they come up during your sleep window, use stimulus control or relaxation strategies	
Worries or problems: List what might come up while you try for sleep	**Solutions or coping strategies:** 2-3 ways to solve or cope with each worry or problem	**Action plan:** After considering pro's and con's for each option, decide on what you will do

Fig. 1.7 This worksheet is an example of what Dr. Medalie uses in clinic to teach patients to get all of their worry thoughts out of their head, and onto paper, well in advance of their sleep window. Printing and use of this handout is not permitted unless directly approved by Dr. Medalie. If interested in accumulating BSM hours or referring patients, Dr. Medalie might be able to help—https:// drlullaby.com/

1.5.3 Worry-time Reading List

Behar E, DiMarco ID, Hekler EB, et al. (2009). Current theoretical models of generalized anxiety disorder (GAD): conceptual review and treatment implications. *J Anxiety Disord. Dec;23*(8):1011–23.

Mobach L, van Schie HT, & Näring GWB (2016). Application of a worry reduction intervention in a medically unexplained symptoms-analogue student-sample. *Psychol Health. Jun;34*(6):677–694.

Versluis A, Verkuil B, & Brosschot JF (2016). Reducing worry and subjective health complaints: A randomized trial of an internet-delivered worry postponement intervention. *Br J Health Psychol. May;21*(2):318–35.

Wahlund T, Mataix-Cols D, Olofsdotter Lauri K, et al. (2021). Brief Online Cognitive Behavioural Intervention for Dysfunctional Worry Related to the COVID-19 Pandemic: A Randomised Controlled Trial. *Psychother Psychosom; 90*(3):191–199.

1.6   Visit 5: Identifying Cognitive Errors

This section reviews a script example, worksheet and references pertaining to the teaching of identification of cognitive errors.

1.6.1 Identifying Cognitive Errors Clinic Talking Points

- Today we will introduce the underpinnings of Aaron Beck's cognitive theory—he taught us that how we think, impacts how we feel and what we do and such factors all interact and impact each other—this concept is referred to as the "Cognitive Triad" and is often seen as a triangle showing the reciprocal relationship between thoughts, feelings and behaviors
- To further focus on changing how we think, there are 3 C's to be aware of: "Catch it, Check it, and Change it"
- We must first be able to identify that we are engaging in a cognitive error to be able to change it, and then in turn have an impact on how we feel and what we do
- Everyone at some point engages in cognitive errors, it is just part of the "human condition"!
- It can be difficult to know when you are having a thought error
- It is typically easiest to notice that you are engaging in a thought error, but realizing that you might have an extended emotional response or overly intense emotional response
- We must expect to feel negative emotions as they are also normal for the "human condition"—the problem is when you have a negative emotion for an extended period, or intensified fashion, that perhaps outweighs what might have expected for the event or interaction

- When that happens, we want you to take a step back and try to identify—what are you truly saying to yourself or about the situation that could perhaps be *overly* negative or exaggerated—that is likely your cognitive error
- These do not have to be about sleep, but certainly can be, you might consider what thoughts you had about sleep the night before, or during the day when you feel tired—there might be a cognitive error there as well
- Once you have identified the cognitive error, we want you to write or type it in the worksheet, then look at the list of "common cognitive errors" and try your best to label your thought according to this list
- This first step is a great way to help create a distance between you and your thoughts and starts you on your journey to learn how to catch it and check it—next visit we will go through how to change it
- We do not want you writing or typing anything during the night—this is just for reflective thought errors or thoughts that arise while awake

1.6.2   Identifying Cognitive Errors Patient Handouts

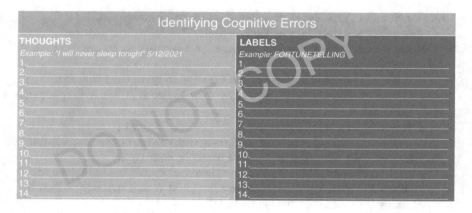

Fig. 1.8   This is an example of a worksheet that Dr. Medalie uses in clinic to teach patients how to track their thought errors and label them according to the list of common cognitive errors. Printing and use of this handout is not permitted unless directly approved by Dr. Medalie. If interested in accumulating BSM hours or referring patients, Dr. Medalie might be able to help—https://drlul-laby.com/

1.6.3   Common Cognitive Errors

1. Overgeneralizing: Believing something will always happen because it happened once before.
   a. Example: Having one bad night of sleep and thinking "I will always have this problem".
2. Fortune-telling: Believing you can predict what will happen in the future, while ignoring other possible outcomes.
   a. Example: I will have trouble sleeping tomorrow night because I have a presentation the following day.
3. Magnifying (Catastrophizing) or Minimizing: Exaggerating the importance of the positive or negative aspects of something.
   a. Example: "This sleep problem is ruining my life" or "Drinking alcohol to fall asleep is not impacting my sleep."
4. Discounting the Positive: Ignoring the good things that happen because you think it must not be important.
   a. Example: "Last night I slept well, but that didn't count because I was exhausted."
5. All-or-Nothing Thinking: Putting things into extreme categories.
   a. Example: "My sleep is completely terrible.".".
6. Jumping to conclusions: Reading the situation a certain way before you have all of the information.
   a. Example: "He's busy because he doesn't want to spend time with me."
7. Mind Reading: Thinking that you can tell how someone else is feeling or what they are thinking.
   a. Example: "They think I'm stupid."
8. Personalization: Taking blame for something that you are not responsible for.
   a. Example: "If I was a better friend he would be doing well."
9. "Should" Statements: Thinking that you should or should not have done something instead of thinking you would have preferred to do something differently.
   a. Example: "I shouldn't have ignored her."

1.6.4   Identifying Cognitive Errors Questionnaire

Dysfunctional Beliefs and Attitudes about Sleep Scale 16 item - Morin, 2007
16 Item, dysfunctional beliefs, expectations and attitudes about sleep
   Name: _____   Date: _____

Dysfunctional Beliefs and Attitudes about Sleep Scale

Several statements reflecting people's beliefs and attitudes about sleep are listed below. Please indicate to what extent you personally agree or disagree with each statement. There is no right or wrong answer. For each statement, circle the number that corresponds to your own *personal belief*. Please respond to all items even though some may not apply directly to your own situation.

		Strongly Disagree - Strongly Agree
1)	I need 8 hours of sleep to feel refreshed and function well during the day.	1 2 3 4 5 6 7 8 9 10
2)	When I don't get the proper amount of sleep on a given night, I need to catch up on the next day by napping or on the next night by sleeping longer.	1 2 3 4 5 6 7 8 9 10
3)	I am concerned that chronic insomnia may have serious consequences on my physical health.	1 2 3 4 5 6 7 8 9 10
4)	I am worried that I may lose control over my abilities to sleep.	1 2 3 4 5 6 7 8 9 10
5)	After a poor night's sleep, I know that it will interfere with my daily activities on the next day.	1 2 3 4 5 6 7 8 9 10
6)	In order to be alert and function well during the day, I believe I would be better off taking a sleeping pill rather than having a poor night's sleep.	1 2 3 4 5 6 7 8 9 10
7)	When I feel irritable, depressed, or anxious during the day, it is mostly because I did not sleep well the night before.	1 2 3 4 5 6 7 8 9 10
8)	When I sleep poorly on one night, I know it will disturb my sleep schedule for the whole week.	1 2 3 4 5 6 7 8 9 10
9)	Without an adequate night's sleep, I can hardly function the next day.	1 2 3 4 5 6 7 8 9 10
10)	I can't ever predict whether I'll have a good or poor night's sleep.	1 2 3 4 5 6 7 8 9 10
11)	I have little ability to manage the negative consequences of disturbed sleep.	1 2 3 4 5 6 7 8 9 10
12)	When I feel tired, have no energy, or just seem not to function well during the day, it is generally because I did not sleep well the night before.	1 2 3 4 5 6 7 8 9 10
13)	I believe insomnia is essentially the result of a chemical imbalance.	1 2 3 4 5 6 7 8 9 10
14)	I feel insomnia is ruining my ability to enjoy life and prevents me from doing what I want.	1 2 3 4 5 6 7 8 9 10
15)	Medication is probably the only solution to my sleeplessness.	1 2 3 4 5 6 7 8 9 10
16)	I avoid or cancel obligations (social, family) after a poor night's sleep.	1 2 3 4 5 6 7 8 9 10

Fig. 1.9 This is research-validated scale commonly used to assess for sleep-related cognitive errors

1.7   Visit 6: Cognitive Restructuring

We review the approach that a Behavioral Sleep Medicine specialist might use to teach cognitive restructuring to patients with insomnia in this section.

1.7.1   Cognitive Restructuring Clinic Talking Points

- Today I will teach you how to go through our cognitive restructuring worksheet using one of your examples
- As you can see there are several columns listed [integrate an example from them while going through each column]
- **Trigger**: Here you will put down what triggered you to have the negative thought—an interaction with someone, waking up during the night, feeling tired during the day, etc.
- **Thought/Label:** For this column, you will put down the thought you had and the label that you would use to categorize what type of thought this is—make sure you are going "deep enough" here so you really get under the hood of the car and identify the darkest part of what you are really saying to yourself or about the situation

- **Emotion/Percent:** This is where you will put down what type of emotional response you had and how intense it was—where 0% is there is none of that emotion present and 100% means you were completely consumed with that emotion—we want to know how intense it was during the darkest point of having this thought –
- **Supporting Facts:** This column is where we want to you transition from being emotional about this topic and get logical—like you are in a court case as a lawyer and you want to just present the facts—you will list the facts that support why this thought would be true. We want you to stay away from opinions or emotions here. Just historical data, frequency of experience, percentage of times this has happened before, etc.
- **Disputing Facts:** Then you will list out the facts disputing the accuracy of this statement- based on your past experience, or what is known and established, what facts dispute the accuracy of this statement.
- **Replacement Thought:** Next you will review the facts supporting the truth of the statement, and the facts disputing the accuracy of this statement—and come up with something more grounded. We do not want you to be overly "rose-tinted" or unrealistic—but just simply summarize what is true. If you were talking to a close friend or family member, how could you more factually reframe this?
- **Emotion/Percent:** Now, we want to you put down the emotion you have when you say this replacement thought to yourself and the intensity of the emotion
- We do not expect that through this process, you will have no negative emotion, but we hope you can see how it might be easier to sleep if ___% of you feels ___ compared to __% of you feeling __.
- We want you to use this exercise during the day at a time when you are experiencing an extreme emotional reaction and struggling with a thought error
- You can also use it reflectively if you recall an intense emotion or negative thought from the previous night or earlier in the day
- If an intense emotion or negative thought comes up while trying for sleep, use stimulus control or relaxation strategies

1.7.2 Cognitive Restructuring Patient Handout

Cognitive Restructuring Worksheet

Triggering moment	Thought and Label	Emotion and % intensity	Supporting Facts	Disputing Facts	Replacement Thought	Emotion and % intensity

Fig. 1.10 This worksheet is an example of what Dr. Medalie uses in clinic with insomnia patients to teach the process of cognitive restructuring. Printing and use of this handout is not permitted unless directly approved by Dr. Medalie. If interested in accumulating BSM hours or referring patients, Dr. Medalie might be able to help—https://drlullaby.com/

1.7.3   Cognitive Restructuring Reading List

Burns, D. (1999). *Feeling good: the new mood therapy.* Rev. and updated. New York: Avon Books.

Clark, D. A. (2013). *Cognitive restructuring. The Wiley handbook of cognitive behavioral therapy.* Wiley. (ch. 2).

Meltzer, L.J., & McLaughlin Crabtree, V. (2015). *Pediatric sleep problems: A clinician's guide to behavioral interventions.* American Psychological Association.

Stallard, P. (2018). *Think good, feel good: a cognitive behavioural therapy workbook for children and young people, second edition.* John Wiley & Sons.

Wolgast, M., Lundh, L.-G., & Viborg, G. (2013). Cognitive restructuring and acceptance: An empirically grounded conceptual analysis. Cognitive Therapy and Research, 37(2), 340–351.

1.8   Visit 7: Maintenance and Relapse Prevention

This section includes a script example, worksheet and references pertaining to the teaching of maintenance and relapse prevention for insomnia patients.

1.8.1   Maintenance and Relapse Prevention Clinic Talking Points

- Today we will start by reviewing data from your first visit compared to your most recent visits
- As you can see, at the start of treatment you were ____, and now you ____.
- While it is great to see this progress, we do know that those with a history of insomnia tend to be vulnerable to a relapse of insomnia
- Looking back at your intake note, given that your precipitating events were ____, a potential trigger for relapse could be if something similar occurs in your future.
- Please share with me any thoughts on what might additionally contribute to a relapse of your insomnia—let's use your worksheet to list these out together and come up with action plans to try and address these potential relapse triggers
- Another important part of today's visit is to emphasize maintenance of the approach you are currently utilizing to sustain gains—of the techniques and strategies we have reviewed throughout CBT-I, which of the changes have been most helpful? Let's list those out with reminders about how you use them and why they have helped—this will help keep you motivated to maintain these changes

- Also, just know that with improvements, it is common to see people start to get less strict about their sleep approach—for example, you might find it reasonable to sleep in by 1 h on weekends instead of keeping your exact waketime from weekdays; or maybe you will stop being as strict about keeping sleep logs
- If you have a relapse—defined as 3 or more nights within a week where you are again struggling with sleep—at that point, you will again want to go back to being super strict about your approach and go back through our worksheets
- You are also always welcome to return to clinic
- We just ask that if you do come back, you have a sleep log completed from the week prior

1.8.2 Maintenance and Relapse Prevention Patient Handout

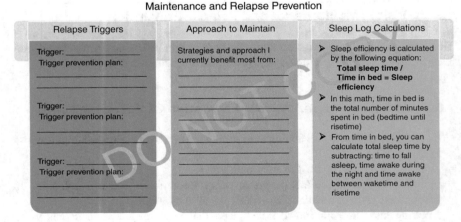

Fig. 1.11 This is a worksheet example of what Dr. Medalie uses teach patients how to maintain CBT-I gains and prevent relapse of insomnia. Printing and use of this handout is not permitted unless directly approved by Dr. Medalie. If interested in accumulating BSM hours or referring patients, Dr. Medalie might be able to help—https://drlullaby.com/

Bibliography

1. American Academy of Sleep Medicine. International classification of sleep disorders. 3rd ed. Darien, IL: American Academy of Sleep Medicine; 2014. p. 21–2.
2. American Academy of Sleep Medicine. International classification of sleep disorders. 3rd ed. Darien, IL: American Academy of Sleep Medicine; 2014. p. 41–2.
3. American Academy of Sleep Medicine. International classification of sleep disorders, vol. 46. 3rd ed. Darien, IL: American Academy of Sleep Medicine; 2014.
4. Morin CM, Vallières A, Ivers H. Dysfunctional beliefs and attitudes about sleep (DBAS): validation of a brief version (DBAS-16). Sleep. 2007;30(11):1547–54.
5. Morin CM, Belleville G, Bélanger L, Ivers H. The insomnia severity index: psychometric indicators to detect insomnia cases and evaluate treatment response. Sleep. 2011;34(5):601–8.

Pediatric Behavioral Sleep Medicine

2

2.1 Visit 1: Intake and Sleep Hygiene

This section shows the process for the first visit in management of pediatric sleep complaints. Our "Visit 1" typically entails a thorough assessment of the presenting complaints, sleep history, psychiatric and medical history, medication review and conceptualization of the diagnosis and plans for treatment. We also review tips for improving sleep hygiene during Visit 1, without describing any interventions that might bias our baseline data collection.

2.1.1 Provider Intake Form

This intake form is an example of what can be used to take notes during a first visit assessing pediatric insomnia complaints.

Note additional data might be warranted for certain CPT codes—the content below only supports the data collection for case conceptualization of an insomnia patient (e.g., psychiatric diagnostic evaluation without medical services 90791 also warrants mental status evaluation)

PEDIATRIC INSOMNIA INTAKE FORM	
Demographic	Patient Name: *** DOB: *** Age: *** Gender: *** Address: *** Phone: *** Email: ***
Sleep symptoms	
Current sleep symptoms	Brief description: *** Frequency: *** Onset: ***

© The Author(s), under exclusive license to Springer Nature Switzerland AG 2022
L. Medalie, *Behavioral Sleep Medicine*,
https://doi.org/10.1007/978-3-031-12574-4_2

PEDIATRIC INSOMNIA INTAKE FORM	
Sleep schedule	Bedtime: ***
	Length of time to fall asleep: ***
	Parent involvement with sleep: ***
	Number of awakenings: ***
	Duration of awakenings: ***
	Parent involvement with sleep: ***
	Waketime: ***
	Out of bed: ***
	Nap time/duration: ***
3 P's	Predisposing factors: ***
	Precipitating events: ***
	Perpetuating factors: ***
Sleep medication	Current medications (OTC or prescribed): ***
	Frequency of use: ***
	When started: ***
	Previous medications tried: ***
Sleep hygiene	Sleep location (parents' bed, their bed): ***
	Electronics (in bedroom, access during the night): ***
	White noise: ***
	Light: ***
	Toy access in bedroom: ***
	Sibling disruption: ***
	Bedtime buddy: ***
	(TEEN) Caffeine: ***
	(TEEN) Alcohol: ***
	(TEEN) Marijuana: ***
	(TEEN) Nicotine: ***
Medically based sleep symptoms	Previous sleep study findings: ***
	Sleep apnea symptoms: ***
	Restless leg symptoms: ***
	Narcolepsy symptoms: ***
	Parasomnias: ***
Psychiatric	
Current mental health symptoms/diagnoses	***
Therapy—current therapy, hospitalization history, therapy history/ experience	***
Medication—current mood medications, history of medications	***
Medical	
Medical diagnoses/ physical symptoms	***
Birth history/ development	***
Current Medications— particular emphasis on medications contributing to insomnia or EDS	***
Impressions/plan	
Diagnosis	***
Treatment goals	***
Treatment plan/referrals	***

2.1.2   Pediatric Sleep Hygiene Clinic Talking Points

- A pre-sleep ritual is an essential part of the sleep hygiene for babies and children
- It is very challenging to go immediately from the stimulation of the day to sleep onset
- Children need 1 h to effectively lower the somatic arousal system and get "sleep ready"
- First, we suggest setting a firm "screens-off" time 1 h before bedtime
- During this hour, we suggest picking an instrumental song and playing it on repeat
- Then start a hot bath
- The final step can either be reading a book (ideally the same book) or singing a song (for babies)
- We also suggest removing all screens from the bedroom completely (as well as toys if possible)—this is called a bedroom sweep
- We encourage use of a white noise machine from bedtime to wake-time for all ages
- When siblings share a bedroom, it helps to use "scattered bedtimes" the older child typically goes to bed 30–60 min after the younger child
- We also suggest making sure kids get enough exercise during the day—exercise supports optimal sleep

For babies:

- The approach to feeding is an essential part of a sleep plan—by 6 months, the need for feeds during the night is rarely present
- We must separate feeds from sleep to succeed with a sleep plan
- The final feed should ultimately be 30–60 min before bedtime, and there should be no calories ingested from bedtime until waketime
- To remove feeds, you can either take an abrupt or gradual (slowly add more water, less milk) depending on what is best for your family

The Figs. 2.1, 2.2, 2.3, 2.4, 2.5 and 2.6, patient handouts, clinic talking points, and diagnostic criteria are shown below to help with the understanding and working with Pediatric Behavioral Sleep Medicine.

2.1.3   Pediatric Sleep Hygiene Handout

This is an example of a handout that Dr. Medalie provides her families at the culmination of a first visit.

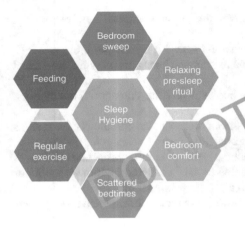

Bedroom sweep: Remove all electronics and toys from the bedroom

Relaxing pre-sleep ritual: Same song on repeat, hot bath, book/sing song

Bedroom comfort: Bedtime buddy, white noise, blackout shades

Scattered bedtimes: Older siblings typically go to bed 30-60 minutes after the younger sibling for shared bedrooms

Regular exercise: Minimize exercise within 3 hours of bedtime

Feeding: Most babies do not need feeds after 6 months – work towards extinguishing the relationship between sleep and feeds

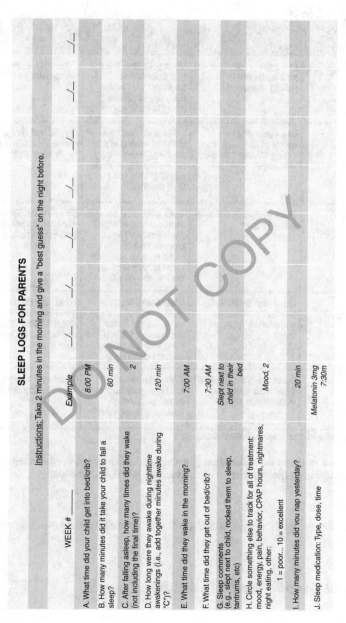

Fig. 2.1 This sleep log is an example of what Dr. Medalie used in clinics to keep track of perceived insomnia symptoms in children during behavioral treatment. Printing and use of this handout is not permitted unless directly approved by Dr. Medalie. If interested in accumulating BSM hours or referring patients, Dr. Medalie might be able to help—https://drlullaby.com/

2.1.4 Pediatric Sleep Log for Parents

BEARS

	TODDLER/PRESCHOOL (2-5 YEARS) (P)	SCHOOL-AGED (6-12 YEARS)	ADOLESCENT (13-18 YEARS)
BEDTIME PROBLEMS	Does your child have any problems going to bed? Falling asleep?	Does your child have any problems at bedtime? (P) Do you have any problems going to bed? (C)	Do you have any problems falling asleep at bedtime? (C)
EXCESSIVE DAYTIME SLEEPINESS	Does your child seem overtired or sleepy a lot during the day? Do they take naps?	Does your child have difficulty waking in the morning, seem sleepy during the day or take naps? (P) Do you feel tired a lot? (C)	Do you feel sleepy a lot during the day? In school? While driving? (C)
AWAKENING DURING THE NIGHT	Does your child wake up a lot at night?	Does your child seem to wake up a lot at night? Any sleepwalking or nightmares? (P) Do you wake up a lot at night? Have trouble getting back to sleep? (C)	Do you wake up a lot at night? Have trouble getting back to sleep? (C)
REGULATORY AND DURATION OF SLEEP	Does your child have a regular bedtime and wake time? What are they?	What time does your child go to bed and get up on school days? Weekends? Do you think they are getting enough sleep? (P)	What time do you usually go to bed on school nights? Weekends? How much sleep do you usually get? (C)
SNORING	Does your child snore a lot or have difficulties breathing at night?	Does your child have loud or nightly snoring or any difficulties breathing at night? (P)	Does your tenager snore loudly or nightly? (P)

(P) Parent-directed question (C) Child-directed question

Fig. 2.2 This is a validated scale that is used by many pediatricians and sleep specialists to get a brief sense of whether sleep symptoms are present in the child they are treating

If kids are old enough to complete sleep logs themselves, they can use the adult logs above

2.1.5 Brief Sleep Screen for Pediatrics

2.1.6 Provider Notes Regarding Pediatric Treatment Plans

This section includes a variety of evidence-based behavioral strategies. Depending on the age group and type of sleep problem reported, different sessions will apply. The previous chapter on Cognitive Behavioral Treatment for Insomnia (CBT-I) will apply to certain older children and teens. A later chapter on Delayed Sleep Phase Syndrome (DSPS) will apply to certain teens.

Your Board-Certified Behavioral Sleep Medicine Supervisor will teach you will strategy to use when, and when CBT-I or DSPS treatment is warranted. Supervision is an essential part of learning how to select appropriate Behavioral Sleep Medicine Treatment Plans, particularly for pediatric insomnia.

For a list of current supervisors, please utilize the Society for Behavioral Sleep Medicine resources.

2.2 Pediatric Follow-up: Learning Independent Sleep

2.2.1 Standard and Graduated Extinction Clinic Talking Points

- First, we need to decide whether we will utilize the standard or graduated extinction method
- Both are considered "evidence-based" and shown in research to be effective methods for removing parent involvement from sleep and reducing nighttime awakenings
- Standard extinction is essentially "cry it out" or abruptly removing your involvement—it typically takes 7–10 nights but can be challenging as the crying or tantrums can be more extreme than you have ever seen, and very hard to tolerate
- The graduated extinction protocol is typically 2–3 weeks long and involves a slower approach to removing parent involvement with sleep
- Now that we have decided on a plan, let's go through the handouts and review the steps you will take from home…let's talk through any customizations based on the unique needs of your family…
- We now need to identify who will take the lead with these steps -we typically suggest the "less attached" parent who is more likely to adhere, takes the lead in implementing the protocol
- We expect this process to be challenging, so please be prepared by making sure you manage stress overall, access peer support, and try your best to stay motivated

2.2.2   Standard Extinction Parent Handout

Standard Extinction Reminders

1. Consistent nightly pre-sleep ritual leading into bedtime: play bedtime song on repeat, bath, book or sing song

2. Holding and cuddling should be at the start of the pre–sleep ritual and less holding and cuddling should be towards the end.

3. Put child into the crib, or have them get into bed, awake but drowsy.

4. Parents leave the bedroom immediately after (while they are still awake).

5. Parents stay out of the bedroom - use headphones, read, and stay distracted.

6. Use a video monitor for ensuring safety.

7. Ignore all crying and tantrums - give your child the time to learn to calm themselves in order to develop self-soothing skills.

8. The crying and screaming will get louder and for longer on initial nights when crying is ignored.

9. When the crying gets louder and for longer, it becomes even more important to ignore the crying otherwise you teach your child that louder crying gets your response and louder crying gets reinforced (i.e., more likely to happen again).

10. Some parents elect to set a "cap" on how much crying they can tolerate. For example, if they wish to use standard extinction but know they would never be able to tolerate more than 1 hour of crying, they go in after 1 hour.

11. If a cap is used, parents should walk in, show their face for under 1-2 minutes and gently state "go to sleep" and walk out.

12. If parents can avoid use of a cap, the approach is treatment is likely to be completed in a shorter timeframe (i.e., less nights of crying).

13. Consistency and sticking to the plan is the most important part of this (and all) strategies.

14. If more than one caregiver is involved, both parents need to both discuss and agree to proceed with the plan.

15. Parents can expect a guilt response to hearing the crying - it is important to remember that letting your child learn to self-soothe is in the best interest of your child

Fig. 2.3 This handout is an example of what Dr. Medalie sends home with parents who elected to try the standard extinction protocol. Printing and use of this handout is not permitted unless directly approved by Dr. Medalie. If interested in accumulating BSM hours or referring patients, Dr. Medalie might be able to help—https://drlullaby.com/

2.2.3 Graduated Extinction Parent Handouts

These handouts are examples of what Dr. Medalie sends home with patients who elected to try the graduated extinction protocol.

Graduated Extinction - BED

Phase I: Camping Out
- ❑ 2 nights – laying next to child in their bed while they fall asleep and return to sleep
- ❑ 2 nights – sitting up at the head of the bed...
- ❑ 2 nights – sitting up on the foot of the bed...
- ❑ 2 nights – sitting in a chair next to the bed...
- ❑ 2 nights – chair in the middle of the room...
- ❑ 2 nights – chair by the door...

Phase I: Scheduled Checks
- ❑ 2 nights – pop your head in every 5 minutes [under 1 min, show your face, stay by the door and ONLY state "I'll be back soon" then walk out] after bedtime *and* each nighttime awakening
- ❑ 2 nights – pop your head in every 10 minutes...
- ❑ 2 nights – pop your head in every 20 minutes...
- ❑ 2 nights – pop your head in every 30 minutes...
- ❑ 2 nights – pop your head in every 40 minutes...

Graduated Extinction - CRIB

Phase I: Camping Out
- ❑ 2 nights – stand next to crib rubbing their arm/hand, while they fall asleep and return to sleep
- ❑ 2 nights – stand next to crib with no contact...
- ❑ 2 nights – sit in a chair next to crib...
- ❑ 2 nights – chair in the middle of the room...
- ❑ 2 nights – chair by the door...

Phase II: Scheduled Checks
- ❑ 2 nights – pop your head on every 5 minutes [under 1 min, show your face, stay by the door and ONLY state "I'll be back soon" then walk out] after bedtime *and* each nighttime awakening
- ❑ 2 nights – pop your head in every 10 minutes...
- ❑ 2 nights – pop your head in every 20 minutes...
- ❑ 2 nights – pop your head in every 30 minutes...
- ❑ 2 nights – pop your head in every 40 minutes...

Printing and use of this handout is not permitted unless directly approved by Dr. Medalie. If interested in accumulating BSM hours or referring patients, Dr. Medalie might be able to help—https://drlullaby.com/

2.2.4 Standard and Graduated Extinction Reading List

No authors listed (2020). 'Cry It Out' Sleep Training Gets Support. *Am J Nurs. Jun;120*(6):15.

Fenton K, Marvicsin D, & Danford CA (2014). An integrative review of sleep interventions and related clinical implications for obesity treatment in children. *J Pediatr Nurs. Nov-Dec;29*(6):503–10.

France, K. G. (2011). *Extinction with parental presence. In Behavioral Treatments for Sleep Disorders* (pp. 275–283). Elsevier.

Gradisar, M., Jackson, K., Spurrier, N. J., et al. (2016). Behavioral interventions for infant sleep problems: A randomized controlled trial. *Pediatrics, 137(6)*, e20151486.

Kahn M, Livne-Karp E, Juda-Hanael M, et al. (2020). Behavioral interventions for infant sleep problems: the role of parental cry tolerance and sleep-related cognitions. *J Clin Sleep Med. Aug 15;16*(8):1275–1283.

Kuhn, B. (2011). The Excuse-Me Drill: A Behavioral Protocol to Promote Independent Sleep Initiation Skills and Reduce Bedtime Problems in Young Children. *In Behavioral Treatments for Sleep Disorders* (pp. 299–309). Elsevier Inc.

Meltzer, L.J., & McLaughlin Crabtree, V. (2015). *Pediatric sleep problems: A clinician's guide to behavioral interventions.* American Psychological Association.

Meltzer, L. J., & Mindell, J. A. (2014). Systematic review and meta-analysis of behavioral interventions for pediatric insomnia. *Journal of Pediatric Psychology, 39*(8), 932–948.

Morgenthaler, T., I., Owens, J., Alessi C, Boehlecke, B., et al. (2006). Practice parameters for behavioral treatment of bedtime problems and night wakings in infants and young children. *Sleep. 29*(10), 1277–1281.

Schenker MT, Ney LJ, Miller LN, et al. (2021). Sleep and fear conditioning, extinction learning and extinction recall: A systematic review and meta-analysis of polysomnographic findings. *Sleep Med Rev. Oct;59*:101501.

Schwichtenberg AJ, Abel EA, Keys E, et al. (2019). Diversity in pediatric behavioral sleep intervention studies. *Sleep Med Rev. Oct*;47:103–111.

Shaughnessy AF (2016). Getting an Infant to Sleep: Graduated Extinction and Sleep Fading are Effective. Am Fam Physician. Nov 1;94(9):750.

Snyder DM, Goodlin-Jones BL, Pionk MJ, et al. (2008). Inconsolable night-time awakening: beyond night terrors. *J Dev Behav Pediatr. Aug;29*(4):311–4.

Vorster APA & Born J (2018). Wakefulness rather than sleep benefits extinction of an inhibitory operant conditioning memory in Aplysia. *Neurobiol Learn Mem. Nov;155*:306-312.

2.2.5   Bedtime Pass Clinic Talking Points

- To minimize "curtain calls" (when your child repeatedly comes out of bed after bedtime) and visits to parents during the night, the bedtime pass works well
- During the day, sit with your child and color/put stickers on some index cards—these are their "bedtime passes"
- Give your child 1–2 bedtime passes at bedtime
- Remind them that if they want to visit parents during the night, they must give up a pass (the parent gets to keep the pass)
- If they have a pass leftover in the morning, they get to exchange it for something special (e.g., a prize from a dollar store prize box, morning treat, etc.)
- Make sure you track progress either on your sleep logs or using a behavior chart—I'll ask in our next visit how many nights they had a pass leftover in the morning

2.2.6   **Bedtime Pass Parent Handout**

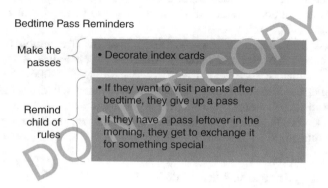

Fig. 2.4 This handout is an example of what Dr. Medalie sends home with families as a reminder of what to do when trying the bedtime pass system. Printing and use of this handout is not permitted unless directly approved by Dr. Medalie. If interested in accumulating BSM hours or referring patients, Dr. Medalie might be able to help—https://drlullaby.com/

2.2.7   Bedtime Pass Reading List

Friman, P. C., Hoff, K. E., Schnoes, C., et al. (1999). The bedtime pass: An approach to bedtime crying and leaving the room. *Archives of Pediatrics & Adolescent Medicine, 153*(10), 1027.

Meltzer, L.J., & McLaughlin Crabtree, V. (2015). Pediatric sleep problems: A clinician's guide to behavioral interventions. American Psychological Association.

Moore, B. A., Friman, P. C., Fruzzetti, A. E., & MacAleese, K. (2006). Brief report: Evaluating the bedtime pass program for child resistance to bedtime--a randomized, controlled trial. *Journal of Pediatric Psychology, 32*(3), 283–287.

Schnoes, C. J. (2017). *The Bedtime Pass. In Behavioral Treatments for Sleep Disorders* (pp. 55–59). Elsevier.

2.2.8   Evening Schedule Clinic Talking Points

- Keeping a structured evening schedule is an essential part of improving sleep in children
- We suggest working with us to outline a specific step-by-step schedule to keep and using cell phone alarms to keep the family on track with the plan
- What time does everyone arrive home?
- What time is dinner?
- What are other activities needed to be completed before bedtime?
- Let's discuss bedtime…
- Let's set the pre-sleep ritual 1 h before bedtime.
- Let's discuss naps (if relevant)
- We'd suggest having a family meeting and making sure everyone is on-board with this schedule
- If so, print it and post it on the refrigerator and do your best to keep the family on track with consistency
- If you fall off track one night, try your best to return to the following night

2.2.9   Evening Schedule Parent Handout

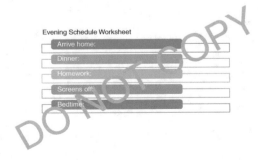

Fig. 2.5 This handout is an example of a tool that Dr. Medalie fills out with families then sends home with them to put up in their home as a reminder to stay on schedule. Printing and use of this handout is not permitted unless directly approved by Dr. Medalie. If interested in accumulating BSM hours or referring patients, Dr. Medalie might be able to help—https://drlullaby.com/

2.2.10 Evening Schedule/Bedtime Routine Reading List

Mindell, J. A., Leichman, E. S., Lee, C., et al. (2017). Implementation of a nightly bedtime routine: How quickly do things improve? *Infant Behavior and Development, 49,* 220–227.

Mindell, J. A., Li, A. M., Sadeh, A., et al. (2015). Bedtime routines for young children: A dose-dependent association with sleep outcomes. *Sleep, 38*(5), 717–722.

Mindell, J. A., Telofski, L. S., Wiegand, B., et al. (2009). A nightly bedtime routine: Impact on sleep in young children and maternal mood. *Sleep, 32*(5), 599–606

Mindell, J. A., & Williamson, A. A. (2018). Benefits of a bedtime routine in young children: Sleep, development, and beyond. *Sleep Medicine Reviews, 40,* 93–108

2.2.11 Behavior Chart Clinic Talking Points

- Many families benefit from using a behavior chart
- The behavior chart can integrate both positive and negative reinforcement
  - Positive reinforcement means that we add a reward to increase the probability of a desired behavior (e.g., pick a prize from a prize box when child got into bed within 5 min of mom saying "bedtime")
  - Negative reinforcement means that we remove a reward to increase the probability of a desired behavior (e.g., remove use of the iPad the next day when child did not get into bed within 5 min of mom saying "bedtime")
- We can use the worksheet to talk through a plan for using the behavior chart
- Let's talk about which target behavior to start with…
- Great, now let's discuss what the reward will be…
- The key to making this work is consistency—if you say that you are going to add or remove a reward contingent on a specific behavior, you must execute, or this will not work

2.2.12 Behavior Chart Clinic Parent Handout

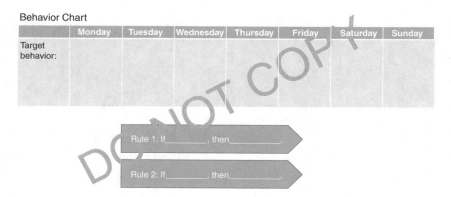

Fig. 2.6 Dr. Medalie uses a tool like this to fill in and send home with families. They can hang this up on their refrigerator or in their child's bedroom to remind everyone of the goal and related reinforcement plan. Printing and use of this handout is not permitted unless directly approved by Dr. Medalie. If interested in accumulating BSM hours or referring patients, Dr. Medalie might be able to help—https://drlullaby.com/

2.2.13 Behavior Chart Reading List

Burke, R. V., Kuhn, B. R., & Peterson, J. L. (2004). Brief report: A "storybook" ending to children's bedtime problems—the use of a rewarding social story to reduce bedtime resistance and frequent night waking. Journal of Pediatric Psychology, 29(5), 389–396

Ivy JW, Meindl JN, Overley E, et al. (2017). Token Economy: A Systematic Review of Procedural Descriptions. *Behav Modif. Sep;41*(5):708-737.

Luersen K, Davis SA, Kaplan SG, et al. (2012). Sticker charts: a method for improving adherence to treatment of chronic diseases in children. *Pediatr Dermatol. Jul-Aug;29*(4):403–8.

McSweeney, F.K., & Murphy, E. S. (2014). The Wiley Blackwell handbook of operant and classical conditioning. John Wiley & Sons. *Chapter 14: Characteristics, Theories, and Implications of Dynamic Changes in Reinforcer Effectiveness.

Meltzer, L.J., & McLaughlin Crabtree, V. (2015). Pediatric sleep problems: A clinician's guide to behavioral interventions. American Psychological Association.

Milby JB. (1975). A review of token economy treatment programs for psychiatric inpatients. *Hosp Community Psychiatry. Oct;26*(10):651–8.

Bibliography

1. American Academy of Sleep Medicine. International classification of sleep disorders 3rd ed (2014). Darien, IL American Academy of Sleep Medicine, 53.
2. Owens JA, Dalzell V. Use of the 'BEARS' sleep screening tool in a pediatric residents' continuity clinic: a pilot study. Sleep Med. 2005;6(1):63–9.
3. Byars KC, Simon SL, Peugh J, Beebe DW. Validation of a brief insomnia severity measure in youth clinically referred for sleep evaluation. J Pediatr Psychol. 2017;42(4):466–75.

Actigraphy

3

3.1   Actigraphy Clinic Talking Points

Set-up

- We will set you up with a wrist-worn device that allows us to collect objective data on your sleep-wake patterns
- You will wear this for 2 weeks 24-h, except if you are submerged in water for 30-min or playing a contact sport
- The watch has an accelerometer built in to infer sleep versus wake based on movement
- There is an "event marker" which is a button on the side—please press this when you get into bed and close your eyes trying for sleep
- Please fill in a sleep log while wearing the watch—make sure to include all nap details

Review [While showing the actogram print-out]

- This is called an actogram—it is a visual depiction of your sleep-wake patterns
- The solid block represents sleep, and the lighter block shows when you are trying for sleep, but awake
- The black vertical lines are your activity counts, higher lines mean higher intensity movement
- The squiggly line is your light exposure
- As you can see, activity and light drop at bedtime and pick back up at waketime
- Based on this data, this suggests... review:
  - Insomnia captured
  - Comment on schedule consistency
  - Mention whether total sleep time seems adequate
  - Comment when there is weeknight sleep loss followed by weekend sleep extension

- Circadian trends
- Napping patterns

The Fig. 3.1 and the clinic talking points are shown to help with the understanding and working with Actigraphy.

3.2 Actogram Example

3.2.1 Actogram

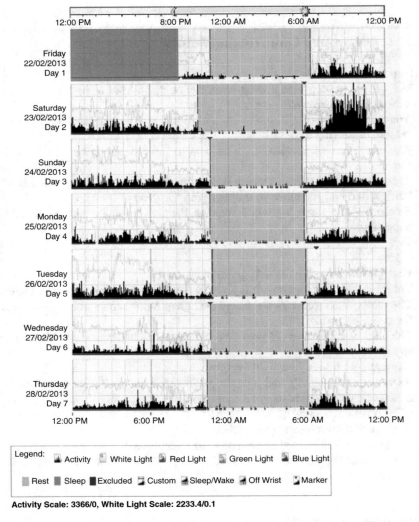

Activity Scale: 3366/0, White Light Scale: 2233.4/0.1

Fig. 3.1 The actogram below is provided to show an example of what a graphic depiction of actigraphy data collection might look like

3.3   Actigraphy Reading List

Aili, K., Åström-Paulsson, S., Stoetzer, U., et al. (2017). Reliability of actigraphy and subjective sleep measurements in adults: The design of sleep assessments. *Journal of Clinical Sleep Medicine, 13*(1), 39–47.

Ancoli-Israel, S. (2009). *Sleep in the Older Adult. In Amlaner,* C. J., Phil, D., & Fuller, P. M. (Eds.). Basics of Sleep Guide (2nd ed., pp. 43-49). Sleep Research Society.

Boulos, M. I., Jairam, T., Kendzerska, T., et al. (2019). Normal polysomnography parameters in healthy adults: a systematic review and meta-analysis. *The Lancet Respiratory Medicine, 7*(6), 533-543.

Hertenstein, E., Gabryelska, A., Spiegelhalder, K., et al. (2018). . Reference data for polysomnography-measured and subjective sleep in healthy adults. *Journal of Clinical Sleep Medicine, 14*(4), 523–532.

Sadeh, A. (2011). The role and validity of actigraphy in sleep medicine: An update. *Sleep Medicine Reviews, 15*, 259-267.

Smith, M. T., McCrae, C. S., Cheung, J., et al. (2018). Use of actigraphy for the evaluation of sleep disorders and circadian rhythm sleep-wake disorders: An american academy of sleep medicine clinical practice guideline. *Journal of Clinical Sleep Medicine, 14*(07), 1231–1237.

Tétreault, É., Bélanger, M.-È., Bernier, A., et al. (2018). Actigraphy data in pediatric research: The role of sleep diaries. *Sleep Medicine, 47*, 86-92.

CBT for CPAP Adherence

4

4.1 Visit 1: Intake and Treatment Planning

This section provides the frequently used talking points, assessment approach and case conceptualization model that Dr. Medalie uses with sleep apnea patients struggling with Positive Airway Pressure (PAP) or Continuous Positive Airway Pressure (CPAP) adherence.

4.1.1 Initial Visit Clinic Talking Points

CPAP Adherence Clinic Talking Points
- I am sorry to hear you are having a hard time with CPAP—this can be very common
- In today's visit, I will go through many questions to get a better sense for what might contribute to this challenge
- I will start by going through questions from our CPAP Adherence intake…
- I appreciate you going through these questions—based on my review, it sounds like your barriers include…
- We will therefore go through roughly __ sessions together so I can support you on your journey to address these barriers
- To get us started, today I will re-review your sleep study results (if available) and go through our Sleep Apnea—CPAP Education Handout
- I am so glad we went through those sleep apnea education points—next I want to remind you of the following sleep hygiene recommendations…
- Finally, let's get you scheduled for your follow-up session—please don't forget to contact the referral suggestions (if appropriate) and complete the CPAP log each morning

4.2 CPAP Intake Form

This form is an example of what Dr. Medalie uses to structure her intake questions with patients struggling to adhere to PAP therapy.

Note additional data might be warranted for certain CPT codes—the content below only supports the data collection for case conceptualization of an insomnia patient (e.g., psychiatric diagnostic evaluation without medical services 90791 also warrants mental status evaluation)

CPAP Adherence—New Patient Note	
Demographic	Patient Name: ***
	DOB: ***
	Age: ***
	Gender: ***
	Address: ***
	Phone: ***
	Email: ***
Sleep symptoms	
Sleep schedule	Bedtime: ***
	Length of time to fall asleep: ***
	(PEDS) Parent involvement with sleep: ***
	Number of awakenings: ***
	Duration of awakenings: ***
	Parent involvement with sleep: ***
	Waketime: ***
	Out of bed: ***
	Nap time/duration: ***
Sleep medication	Current medications (OTC or prescribed): ***
	Frequency of use: ***
	When started: ***
	Previous medications tried: ***
Sleep hygiene	(PEDS) Sleep location (parents' bed, their bed): ***
	Electronics (in bedroom, access during the night): ***
	White noise: ***
	Light: ***
	(PEDS) Toy access in bedroom: ***
	(PEDS) Sibling disruption: ***
	(PEDS) Bedtime buddy: ***
	(ADULT/TEEN) Caffeine: ***
	(ADULT/TEEN) Alcohol: ***
	(ADULT/TEEN) Marijuana: ***
	(ADULT/TEEN) Nicotine: ***
	(ADULT) Partner co-sleeping: ***
Medically-based sleep symptoms	Previous sleep study findings: ***
	Sleep apnea symptoms: ***
	Restless leg symptoms: ***
	Narcolepsy symptoms: ***
	Parasomnias: ***
Psychiatric	
Current mental health symptoms/diagnoses	***

CPAP Adherence—New Patient Note	
Therapy—current therapy, hospitalization history, therapy history/experience	***
Medication—current mood medications, history of medications	***
Medical	
Medical diagnoses/ physical symptoms	***
(PEDS)Birth history/ development	***
Current Medications— particular emphasis on medications contributing to insomnia or EDS	***
CPAP Barriers	
Use the CPAP Adherence Barriers Guide here	
• Knowledge deficiency	
• Interface	
• Pressure	
• Humidifier Settings	
• Insomnia	
• Accidental non-compliance	
• Claustrophobia	
• Motivation	
• Mental health comorbidities	
• Medical comorbidities	
Impressions/plan	
Diagnosis	***
Treatment goals	***
Treatment plan/referrals	***

The Figs. 4.1, 4.2 and 4.3**, patient handouts, clinic talking points, CPAP adherence barriers guide, and diagnostic criteria are shown below to help with the understanding and working with CBT for CPAP Adherence.**

4.2.1 CPAP Adherence Barriers Guide

Dr. Medalie uses this guide to structure barrier assessment questions and conceptualize the underlying reasons for insufficient PAP adherence.

Instructions: Replies to the following questions will be noted in your CPAP Adherence Intake Form. After going through these questions, and reviewing replies in the intake, you can then summarize your treatment plan using the appropriate plans outlined below.

Barrier: Knowledge deficiency

Question: Do you understand why you need to wear CPAP?

Plan:
1. Educate patient using the behavioral strategy—*psychoeducation*—review the CPAP-Sleep Apnea Education Handout
2. Sleep study results: If available, re-review the results of the sleep study

Barrier: Interface

Question: Do you have any issues with mask comfort, straps, equipment, or leak?

Plan: Refer patient to talk to their homecare company/CPAP supplier

Barrier: Pressure

Question: Are you having issues with pressure or high apnea-hypopnea index despite use?

Plan: Refer patient to talk to their MD and evaluate whether pressure adjustments or repeat CPAP titration study is necessary

Ramp reminders: If patient does not have a high apnea-hypopnea index, they might need a reminder about the ramp feature
- When you push the ramp button/set-up the ramp feature, this allows the machine to start with the lowest pressure and gradually work up to the optimal pressure
- If you wake up and try to return to sleep with the optimal pressure (i.e., a high pressure setting), it can lead to insomnia for some patients

Barrier: Humidifier Settings

Question: Is dryness or excess moisture an issue?

Plan: Remind patient about adjusting the humidifier settings—they can increase to higher humidification to address dryness and lower humidification to address excess moisture
- Refer patient to their homecare company to address follow-up questions
- Refer patient for medical support (e.g., ENT, sleep MD or PCP) if persistent congestion is noted as a barrier

Barrier: Insomnia

Question: Are you taking more than 30 min to fall asleep or return to sleep, 3 or more nights per week? Is this causing problems functioning or significant distress?

Plan: Complete 5-8 follow-up sessions—i.e., initiate Cognitive Behavioral Treatment for Insomnia (see previous chapter) while working on any other barriers mentioned

Barrier: Accidental Non-compliance

Question: Are you "accidentally" falling asleep or returning to sleep without CPAP (e.g., falling asleep on the couch watching television, waking up with CPAP on the floor)?

Plan: Complete 2–3 follow-up sessions to support progress addressing such issues:
1. Avoid dozing in the evenings:
   - Recognize earliest signs of dozing (eyes heavy, yawning, head feeling heavy)—stand up and walk around
   - Set an earlier bedtime so that you are in bed before the sleepiness peaks
   - Have family member or spouse support the goal
2. Leave CPAP on during nighttime awakenings:
   - When going to the bathroom, leave the mask on and just un-hook the hose
   - If your bed partner or family member sees you asleep without CPAP, have them gently wake you to encourage putting it back on

Barrier: Claustrophobia

Question: Do you fear tight spaces or being trapped, to the extent where you are avoiding CPAP because of it? Is your anticipation of wearing CPAP producing a fear response?

Plan: Complete 2–4 follow-up sessions to support progress addressing such issues:
1. Desensitization: talk through the handout and follow-up on progress with exposure hierarchy trials
2. Relaxation strategies: use scripting and worksheets provided in the previous chapter—NOTE: patients cannot easily use diaphragmatic breathing while wearing CPAP, but they can use it before putting on CPAP; they can use positive imagery and progressive muscle relaxation while wearing CPAP

Barrier: Motivation

Question: Are you motivated to wear CPAP?

Plan: Complete 2–3 follow-up sessions to support change and improve motivation:
1. Motivational enhancement strategies: use the worksheets with patient to address motivation issues
2. Behavior chart: add rewards the morning after CPAP was worn
3. Support: include family members in a visit to have them support and encourage CPAP adherence

Barrier: Mental health

Question: Are depressive symptoms, anxiety or other mental health challenges/stressors interfering with CPAP adherence?

Plan:
1. Refer to start therapy and/or medication management
2. Psychoeducation: Discuss the relationship between untreated sleep apnea and mood—emphasize the importance of continuing to work on CPAP adherence while working with the psychiatry referral – e.g., the bi-directional relationship of sleep and mood: poor sleep quality increases mood symptoms, and elevated mood symptoms create challenges with sleep

Barrier: Medical comorbidity

Question: Are unmanaged medical symptoms (e.g., pain, allergies, irritable bowel symptoms, etc.) interfering with CPAP adherence?

Plan:
1. Refer to the appropriate medical treatment provider or encourage patient to discuss further with primary care
2. Psychoeducation: Discuss the relationship between untreated sleep apnea and such symptoms—emphasize the importance of continuing to work on CPAP adherence while working with the medical referral—e.g., bi-directional relationship of sleep and pain: poor sleep quality increases pain perception, and elevated pain creates challenges with sleep

4.2.2 Obstructive Sleep Apnea, Adult Diagnostic Criteria

Obstructive Sleep Apnea, Adult

ICD-9-CM code: 327.23   ICD-10-CM code: G47.33

Diagnostic Criteria
(A and B) or C satisfy the criteria

A. The presence of one or more of the following:
   a. The patient complains of sleepiness, nonrestorative sleep, fatigue, or insomnia symptoms.
   b. The patient wakes with breath holding, gasping, or choking.
   c. The bed partner or other observer reports habitual snoring, breathing interruptions, or both during the patient's sleep.
   d. The patient has been diagnosed with hypertension, a mood disorder, cognitive dysfunction, coronary artery disease, stroke, congestive heart failure, atrial fibrillation, or type 2 diabetes, mellitus.
B. Polysomnography (PSG) or OCST demonstrates:
   a. Five or more predominantly obstructive respiratory events (obstructive and mixed apneas, hypopneas, or respiratory effort related arousals [RERAs]) per hour of sleep during PSG or per hour of monitoring (OCST).
      OR
C. PSG or OCST demonstrates:
   a. Fifteen or more predominantly obstructive respiratory events (apneas, hypopneas, or RERAs) per hour of sleep during a PSG or per hour of monitoring (OCST).

4.2.3 Obstructive Sleep Apnea, Pediatric Diagnostic Criteria

Obstructive Sleep Apnea, Pediatric

ICD-9-CM code: 327.23   ICD-10-CM code: G47.33

Diagnostic Criteria
Criteria A and B must be met

A. The presence of one or more of the following:
   a. Snoring.
   b. Labored, paradoxical, or obstructed breathing during the child's sleep.
   c. Sleepiness, hyperactivity, behavioral problems, or learning problems.

B. PSG demonstrates one or both of the following:
  a. One or more obstructive apneas, mixed apneas, or hypopneas, per hour of sleep.
     OR
  b. A pattern of obstructive hypoventilation, defined as at least 25% of total sleep time with hypercapnia ($PaCO_2 > 50$ mm Hg) in association with one or more of the following:
     i.   Snoring.
     ii. Flattening of the inspiratory nasal pressure waveform.
     iii. Paradoxical thoracoabdominal motion.

4.3 CPAP Adherence Patient Handouts

4.3.1 Psychoeducation Patient Handout

Dr. Medalie uses this handout to give to sleep apnea patients at the end of their first visit. They can use this as review on what sleep apnea is, risks if left untreated, and benefits of PAP therapy.

Sleep Apnea-CPAP Education

- **Sleep apnea defined**
  - Most common type: Obstructive sleep apnea
    - A blockage in the airway interferes with adequate airflow
      - Imagine a pinched straw
    - The obstructed airway tells the brain "something is wrong, wake up"
      - This causes sleep fragmentation, which results in daytime sleepiness
    - Drops in oxygen and cardiac rhythm changes can occur alongside these nighttime respiratory events
    - Depending on the number of times per hour someone has these events, they are defined as mild (5-15 times per hour), moderate (16-30 times per hour) or severe (over 30 times per hour)
- **Symptoms of sleep apnea**
  - Excessive daytime sleepiness
  - Snoring that can be heard outside the bedroom
  - Choking or gasping sensations
  - Morning headaches
  - Unfreshing sleep
  - Dry mouth
- **Sleep apnea treatment**
  - The first line treatment recommended for obstructive sleep apnea is positive airway pressure (PAP)
  - Continuous positive airway pressure (CPAP) is the most common type of PAP therapy
  - PAP therapy works by holding the airway open using pressurized air
  - Room air comes through the machine, hose and up through the airway at specific intensity (i.e., CPAP pressure) to prevent the airway blockage and decrease the nighttime respiratory problem

- **Untreated sleep apnea**
  - Obesity risks
    - Increased appetite
    - Difficulty losing weight
  - Medical risks
    - Diabetes
    - Hypertension
    - Heart attack
    - Stroke
  - Psychological risks
    - Depressive symptoms
    - Quality of life Impact
  - Daytime Functioning risks
    - Sleepiness
    - Memory problems
    - Attention lapses
    - Auto accidents

- **Benefits of CPAP**
  Sleep apnea
  - Apnea-hypopnea index
  - Oxyhemoglobin saturation
  - Cortical arousals associated with events
  Daytime results *for some
  - Elevated mood
  - Energy
  - Cognitive function improvement

Printing and use of this handout is not permitted unless directly approved by Dr. Medalie. If interested in accumulating BSM hours or referring patients, Dr. Medalie might be able to help—https://drlullaby.com/

4.4   CPAP Adherence Patient Handouts

4.4.1   Desensitization Patient Handout

CPAP Desensitization Steps

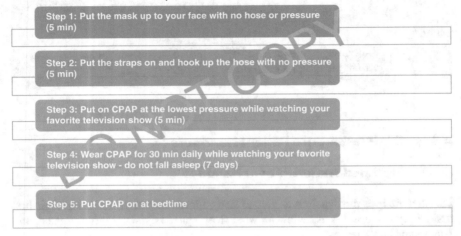

Step 1: Put the mask up to your face with no hose or pressure (5 min)

Step 2: Put the straps on and hook up the hose with no pressure (5 min)

Step 3: Put on CPAP at the lowest pressure while watching your favorite television show (5 min)

Step 4: Wear CPAP for 30 min daily while watching your favorite television show - do not fall asleep (7 days)

Step 5: Put CPAP on at bedtime

Fig. 4.1 This handout is sent home with patients as a reminder of steps to use for desensitization. Printing and use of this handout is not permitted unless directly approved by Dr. Medalie. If interested in accumulating BSM hours or referring patients, Dr. Medalie might be able to help— https://drlullaby.com/

4.5   CPAP Adherence Patient Handouts

4.5.1   Motivational Enhancement Patient Handout

CPAP Motivation Worksheet

• **Motivation rating**
  • How motivated are you to use CPAP on a scale of 0-10? _____
  • What would it take to move you from a_ to a_?

  _____
  _____

• **Values**
  • What do you value most in this world? _____
    • How could treating sleep apnea support what you value?

  _____
  _____

• **Decision**
  • Pros and cons of using CPAP versus not using CPAP

  _____
  _____

Fig. 4.2 Dr. Medalie uses this worksheet with patients in session. She either has sleep apnea patients fill out this form themselves, or asks them questions verbally and sends them home with their completed worksheet as a reminder. Printing and use of this handout is not permitted unless directly approved by Dr. Medalie. If interested in accumulating BSM hours or referring patients, Dr. Medalie might be able to help—https://drlullaby.com/

4.6   CPAP Adherence Patient Handouts

4.6.1   Adherence Tracking

NOTE: Some providers have access to CPAP download data which can either replace or provide a helpful compliment to behavioral data.

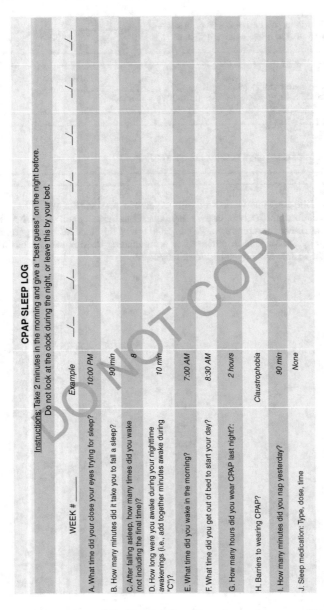

Fig. 4.3 This sleep log is used by Dr. Medalie with patients who are tracking both insomnia symptoms, and their subjective experience of PAP adherence. Printing and use of this handout is not permitted unless directly approved by Dr. Medalie. If interested in accumulating BSM hours or referring patients, Dr. Medalie might be able to help—https://drlullaby.com/

4.6.2 CPAP Adherence Reading List

Aloia MS, Arndt JT, Riggs RL, et al. (2004). Clinical management of poor adherence to CPAP: motivational enhancement. *Behav Sleep Med. 2*(4):205-22.

Bakker JP, Wang R, Weng J, et al. (2016). Motivational Enhancement for Increasing Adherence to CPAP: A Randomized Controlled Trial. *Chest, Aug;150*(2):337-45.

Chernyak Y (2020). Improving CPAP Adherence for Obstructive Sleep Apnea: A Practical Application Primer on CPAP Desensitization. *MedEdPORTAL, Sep 15*;16:10963.

Hawkins, S. M. M., Jensen, E. L., Simon, S. L., et al. (2016). Correlates of pediatric cpap adherence. *Journal of Clinical Sleep Medicine, 12*(06), 879–884.

King, M. S., Xanthopoulos, M. S., & Marcus, C. L. (2014). Improving positive airway pressure adherence in children. *Sleep Medicine Clinics, 9*(2), 219–234.

Lai AYK, Fong DYT, Lam JCM, et al. (2014). The efficacy of a brief motivational enhancement education program on CPAP adherence in OSA: a randomized controlled trial. *Chest, Sep;146*(3):600-610.

Shapiro, G. K., & Shapiro, C. M. (2010). Factors that influence CPAP adherence: An overview. *Sleep and Breathing, 14*(4), 323–335.

Stepnowsky, C., Zamora, T., Edwards, C., et al. (2013). Interventions to improve cpap adherence and outcomes: Role of theory and behavioral change techniques. *Journal of Sleep Disorders & Therapy, 02*(05).

Sweetman A, Lack L, Catcheside PG, et al. (2019). Cognitive and behavioral therapy for insomnia increases the use of continuous positive airway pressure therapy in obstructive sleep apnea participants with comorbid insomnia: a randomized clinical trial. *Sleep, Dec 24;42*(12):zsz178.

Richards D, Bartlett DJ, Wong K, et al. (2007). Increased adherence to CPAP with a group cognitive behavioral treatment intervention: a randomized trial. *Sleep, May;30*(5):635-40.

Weaver TE. Novel Aspects of CPAP Treatment and Interventions to Improve CPAP Adherence. *J Clin Med, Dec 16;8*(12):2220.

Bibliography

1. American Academy of Sleep Medicine. International classification of sleep disorders 3rd (2014). Darien, IL American Academy of Sleep Medicine, 53.
2. American Academy of Sleep Medicine. International classification of sleep disorders 3rd (2014). Darien, IL American Academy of Sleep Medicine, 63.

Imagery Rehearsal Therapy for Nightmare Disorder

5

5.1 Visit 1: Nightmare Intake and Psychoeducation

5.1.1 IRT Introduction Clinic Talking Points

- I am so sorry to hear you are struggling with nightmares
- Today we will spend time going through specific questions so I can better understand your nightmare history, confirm your diagnosis, and establish a treatment plan
- After going through the intake, I will review "Facts about Nightmares" and how to complete our nightmare log
- It's important to know that we do not want you describing the details of your nightmares
- I might ask you to overview the general themes and whether there is repetition, but we do not want you describing the nightmares in detail
- Further, it is best you do not describe the nightmares in detail to friends, family etc
- Robert Stickgold PhD's dream research out of Harvard, has taught us that what we experience and are exposed to during our waking life comes up in our dream content
- Reviewing nightmare detail during your waking life makes you more likely to experience nightmares again the following night
- We are not encouraging avoidance per se, but more so starting to teach you healthy habits to discourage the ongoing pattern of repeating nightmares
- Now I will go through the nightmare intake with you…
- I appreciate you spending time discussing your nightmare history, now I will review nightmare facts and how to use the nightmare log…
- Let's review some sleep hygiene reminders based on what you told me about your sleep habits today
- Our final step today is to remind you to complete the nightmare log each morning and schedule your next visit—Imagery Rehearsal Therapy includes 5 visits total (including today) which are typically completed either weekly or bi-weekly

The Fig. 5.1, **patient handouts, clinic talking points, provider guides, and diagnostic criteria are shown below to help with the understanding and working with Imagery Rehearsal Therapy for Nightmare Disorder.**

5.1.2   Provider Guide to Comorbidities and Differentials

COMORBIDITIES
1. **Insomnia Disorder:**
   Given the frequent overlap between insomnia and nightmares, you will need to decide whether to complete Cognitive Behavioral Treatment for Insomnia before or after Imagery Rehearsal Therapy
   a. If nightmares are "the only reason" the patient has insomnia, it makes sense to start with Imagery Rehearsal Therapy
   b. If insomnia started before nightmares and insomnia is the distress response/functional impact of insomnia is more severe than nightmares, it makes sense to start with Cognitive Behavioral Treatment for Insomnia
   c. If the order is not obvious, consider asking the patient for their preference and consulting with your referring doctor
2. **Post-Traumatic Stress Disorder (PTSD):**
   Typically, patients who meet criteria for Nightmare Disorder report history of trauma and symptoms of PTSD.
   a. If at the time you see patient, they continue to report flashbacks, avoidance behaviors and meet criteria for PTSD, refer them to an anxiety disorders specialist who can initiate evidence-based treatment for PTSD (e.g., Cognitive Processing Therapy (CPT), Prolonged Exposure Therapy and/or Eye Movement Desensitization and Reprocessing (EMDR)
   b. After they complete PTSD treatment, if they continue to meet criteria for Nightmare Disorder, they can then return to see you with a completed nightmare log from the week prior
   c. If they no longer meet criteria for Nightmare Disorder after treating PTSD, they do not need to complete Imagery Rehearsal Therapy

DIFFERENTIALS
1. **Anxious Dreams:**
   Patients often confuse anxious dreams with nightmares, but they are very different symptoms with different treatment implications
   a. Nightmares are often described as "horror movies" and evoke a fear response. They are typically replays of trauma elements
   b. Anxious dreams evoke worry and are often experienced in patients with elevated daytime anxiety. Our primary emotional tone and daytime experience shows up in our dream life. Patients who struggle to control daytime anxiety will have anxious tones to their dreams. Typically, patients with anxious dreams deny history of trauma

    c. If you review the description of nightmares versus anxious dreams and anxious dreams are confirmed, Imagery Rehearsal Therapy might not be warranted. Instead, you may consider referring patient to a psychologist specializing in whichever anxiety disorder they meet criteria for (e.g., a psychologist who can initiate Cognitive Behavioral Therapy for Generalized Anxiety Disorder)

2. **REM Behavior Disorder**

    Patients with REM Behavior Disorder can sometimes be mistaken for Nightmare Disorder. If you are referred a patient diagnosed with Parkinson's Disease or Lew body dementia (or presenting with such symptoms) it is important to clarify this before proceeding with Imagery Rehearsal Therapy.

    a. If patient is kicking and thrashing violently during dream content, that can be a sign or symptom of REM Behavior Disorder. Being male and over 50 years old can be risk factors for REM Behavior Disorder

    b. A helpful differentiating question can be querying whether there is history of trauma and PTSD symptoms. If there is kicking and thrashing during dreams, with no trauma history, a referral to a sleep physician is likely warranted. The sleep physician can screen for REM Behavior Disorder and consider medication management options if appropriate

3. **Sleep terrors**

    Parents who present with concerns pertaining "blood curdling screams", screaming and crying during the night might initially suspect nightmares are occurring.

    a. Night terrors (or night terrors) typically occur during slow wave sleep in the first third of the night. They can be quite terrifying for parents to witness. They are often brief

    b. The easiest way to differentiate nightmares from night terrors is to ask whether patient recalls the events the next day. There is typically no next day recall following night terrors

    c. In addition, children typically do not recognize parents during night terrors and may engage in non-sensical speech

    d. If you learn that these events are night terrors, Imagery Rehearsal Therapy would not be appropriate. Instead see later chapter on Parasomnias to understand next steps for addressing this parasomnia

5.1.3   Imagery Rehearsal Therapy Intake Form

Dr. Medalie uses this form to assess nightmares during the first session of Imagery Rehearsal Therapy (IRT).

    Note additional data might be warranted for certain CPT codes—the content below only supports the data collection for case conceptualization of an insomnia patient (e.g., psychiatric diagnostic evaluation without medical services 90791 also warrants mental status evaluation)

NIGHTMARE INTAKE- New Patient Note

Demographic	Patient Name: ***
	DOB: ***
	Age: ***
	Gender: ***
	Address: ***
	Phone: ***Email: ***
Nightmare symptoms	
Description	Nights per week: ***
	Onset of symptoms: ***
	Theme (without details): ***
	Repetition: ***
	Triggers: ***
	Severity (1-10, where 10 is worst): ***
Comorbidity/ & rule out questions	History of trauma: ***
	Current PTSD symptoms:
	Kicking/thrashing: ***
	Next day recall: ***
Sleep symptoms	
Sleep schedule	Bedtime: ***Length of time to fall asleep: ***
	(PEDS) Parent involvement with sleep: ***
	Number of awakenings: ***
	Duration of awakenings: ***
	Parent involvement with sleep: ***
	Waketime: ***
	Out of bed: ***
	Nap time/duration: ***
Sleep medication	Current medications (OTC or prescribed): ***
	Frequency of use: ***
	When started: ***
	Previous medications tried: ***
Sleep hygiene	(PEDS) Sleep location (parents' bed, their bed): ***Electronics (in bedroom, access during the night): ***
	White noise: ***
	Light: ***
	(PEDS) Toy access in bedroom: ***
	(PEDS) Sibling disruption: ***
	(PEDS) Bedtime buddy: ***
	(ADULT/TEEN) Caffeine: ***
	(ADULT/TEEN) Alcohol: ***
	(ADULT/TEEN) Marijuana: ***
	(ADULT/TEEN) Nicotine: ***
	(ADULT) Partner co-sleeping: ***
Medically based sleep symptoms	Previous sleep study findings: ***
	Sleep apnea symptoms: ***
	Restless leg symptoms: ***
	Narcolepsy symptoms: ***
	Parasomnias: ***
Psychiatric	
Current mental health symptoms/diagnoses	***

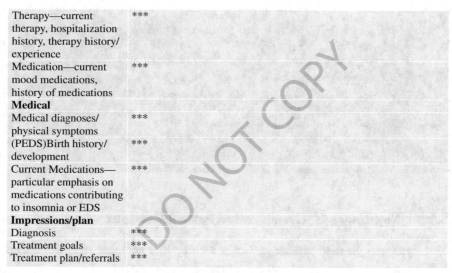

Therapy—current therapy, hospitalization history, therapy history/ experience	***
Medication—current mood medications, history of medications	***
Medical	
Medical diagnoses/ physical symptoms	***
(PEDS)Birth history/ development	***
Current Medications— particular emphasis on medications contributing to insomnia or EDS	***
Impressions/plan	
Diagnosis	***
Treatment goals	***
Treatment plan/referrals	***

Printing and use of this handout is not permitted unless directly approved by Dr. Medalie. If interested in accumulating BSM hours or referring patients, Dr. Medalie might be able to help—https://drlullaby.com/.

5.1.4 Nightmare Disorder Diagnostic Criteria

Nightmare Disorder

ICD-9-CM code: 307.47   ICD-10-CM code: F51.5

Diagnostic Criteria

Criteria A–C must be met

A. Repeated occurrences of extended, extremely dysphoric, and well-remembered dreams that usually involve threats to survival, security, or physical integrity.

B. On awakening from the dysphoric dream, the person rapidly becomes oriented and alert.

C. the dream experience, or the sleep disturbance produced by awakening from it, causes clinically significant distress or impairment in social, occupational, or other important areas of functioning as indicated by the report of at least one of the following:

   a. Mood disturbance (e.g., persistence of nightmare effect, anxiety, dysphoria).

   b. Sleep resistance (e.g., bedtime anxiety, fear of sleep/subsequent nightmares).

    c. Cognitive impairments (e.g., intrusive nightmare imagery, impaired concentration, or memory).

    d. Negative impact on caregiver of family functioning (e.g., nighttime disruption).

    e. Behavioral problems (e.g., bedtime avoidance, fear of the dark).

    f. Daytime sleepiness.

    g. Fatigue or low energy.

    h. Impaired occupational or educational function.

    i. Impaired interpersonal/social function.

5.1.5   Nightmare Psychoeducation Patient Handout

This handout is given to patients to take home after they complete their IRT intake session.

Nightmare Education

REM Sleep and Nightmares:
- Dreams and nightmares typically occur during REM sleep
  - Although short and less vivid dreams can occur in non-REM sleep
- REM is a sleep stage typically marked by "muscle atonia"
  - Muscles except for eyes and diaphragm are paralyzed during REM
- Medication impacting REM sleep can impact nightmare intensity
  - Check with your physician to see if this is relevant
- Alcohol impacts REM sleep and can likewise impact nightmare intensity
  - REM suppression in the first half of the night and REM rebound in the second half of the night after alcohol consumption
- Medical symptoms which impact sleep quality (e.g., sleep apnea, periodic limb movement disorder, pain, allergies, etc) can impact REM sleep
  - Talk to your doctor about such symptoms to ultimately maximize management of nightmares

Trauma and Nightmares:
- Nightmares often occur as a result of trauma
- Initially when trauma first occurs, it is too emotionally devastating to process
  - The brain avoids processing during the day, then instead processes through dreams at night
  - This protective process is initially helpful, but overtime this turns into a "habit"
  - Night after night, the brain gets used to going into nightmare mode and this learned behavior is automated and no longer helpful

- Patients should make sure PTSD treatment is completed before starting Imagery Rehearsal Therapy
  - Many patients continue to have nightmares even after completing PTSD treatment as nightmares can take on a "life of their own"

Treating nightmares:
- Imagery Rehearsal Therapy (IRT) is the recommended treatment for Nightmare Disorder
- Prazosin is a medication which can be used in severe nightmare cases
- IRT is shown to help decrease severity and frequency of nightmares
- When nightmares decrease, total sleep time can therefore increase
- The increased sleep duration resulting from successful IRT can help support mood, cognitive functioning, energy and overall health
- Untreated nightmares can result in sleep avoidance, prolonged nighttime awakenings, and the common risks of sleep loss
  - Irritability/poor frustration tolerance
  - Anxiety and depressive symptoms
  - Low energy
  - Poor concentration
  - Sub-optimal immune system functioning

Printing and use of this handout is not permitted unless directly approved by Dr. Medalie. If interested in accumulating BSM hours or referring patients, Dr. Medalie might be able to help—https://drlullaby.com/.

5.1.6 Imagery Rehearsal Therapy Tracking Form

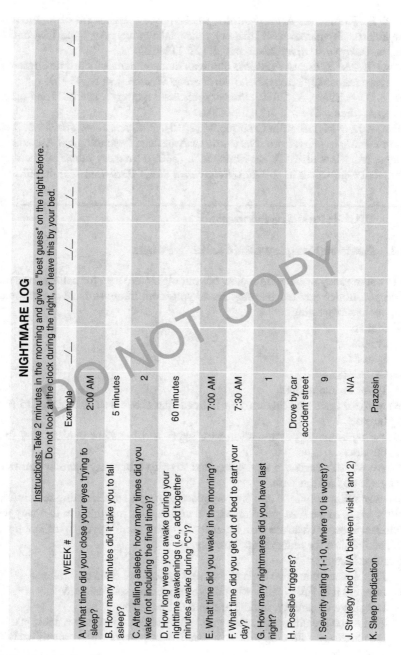

Fig. 5.1 This log is sent home with patients to track nightmare symptoms relevant to IRT, along-side insomnia symptoms. Printing and use of this handout is not permitted unless directly approved by Dr. Medalie. If interested in accumulating BSM hours or referring patients, Dr. Medalie might be able to help—https://drlullaby.com/

5.1.7   Imagery Rehearsal Therapy Reading List

Ellis, T. E., Rufino, K. A., & Nadorff, M. R. (2019). Treatment of nightmares in psychiatric inpatients with imagery rehearsal therapy: An open trial and case series. *Behavioral Sleep Medicine, 17*(2), 112–123.

Krakow, B., & Zadra, A. (2006). Clinical management of chronic nightmares: Imagery rehearsal therapy. *Behavioral Sleep Medicine, 4*(1), 45–70.

Krakow, B., & Zadra, A. (2010). Imagery rehearsal therapy: Principles and practice. *Sleep Medicine Clinics, 5*(2), 289–298.

Meltzer, L.J., & McLaughlin Crabtree, V. (2015). *Pediatric sleep problems: A clinician's guide to behavioral interventions.* American Psychological Association.

St-Onge, M., Mercier, P., & De Koninck, J. (2009). Imagery rehearsal therapy for frequent nightmares in children. *Behavioral Sleep Medicine, 7*(2), 81–98.

5.2   Visit 2: Positive Imagery

5.2.1   Positive Imagery Clinic Talking Points

- Let's start today's visit with review of your nightmare logs for patterns and trends
- Did you notice any triggers that made you more likely to have a nightmare or higher severity rating?
  – Sights
  – Smells
  – Sounds
  – Experiences
  – Types of interactions
- Were there habits or factors you noticed that made you less likely to have a nightmare?
- Please continue to pay attention to triggers and behavior choices that impact nightmares
- Today we will review a strategy called "Positive Imagery" which you may or may not be familiar with
- We teach this technique as a starting place to prepare for learning rescripting
- We want to make sure you can learn to utilize your imagination in a way where you can focus on a scene with intensity in your "mind's eye" to ultimately learn the techniques for reducing nightmares
- Positive imagery:
  – Pick a place you have been to that makes you feel calm and relaxed
  – Imagine it in full detail—what do you see, hear, taste and smell.
  – Imagine a beginning, middle and end to that scene.
  – While you are doing this, your mind will wander, and when it does, just imagine the thought floating off into a cloud, then gently bring yourself back to the calming scene

- For today's homework, we want you to practice positive imagery between now and our next visit
- Either type up your script for the positive imagery scene [some providers do this together with patient in session], or mentally walk yourself through the scene
- A practice session should take about 10-15 minutes
- Practice sessions:
  - During the day after something stressful occurred
  - During the hour before bedtime—relaxing pre-sleep ritual
  - To transition into sleep at the start of the night
  - To transition back to sleep in the middle of the night
- In addition to practicing positive imagery, we want you to continue completing the nightmare logs

5.2.2   Positive Imagery Reading List

Krau DS (2020). The multiple uses of guided imagery. *Nurs Clin North Am, Dec; 55*(4): 467-474.

Nooner AK, Dwyer K, DeShea L, et al. (2016). Using Relaxation and Guided Imagery to Address Pain, Fatigue, and Sleep Disturbances: A Pilot Study. *Clin J Oncol Nurs. Oct 1;20*(5):547-52.

Schmid C, Hansen K, Kröner-Borowik T, et al. (2021). Imagery Rescripting and Imaginal Exposure in Nightmare Disorder Compared to Positive Imagery: A Randomized Controlled Trial. *Psychother Psychosom, 90*(5):328-340.

Waltman SH, Shearer D, & Moore BA (2018). Management of Post-Traumatic Nightmares: a Review of Pharmacologic and Nonpharmacologic Treatments Since 2013. *Curr Psychiatry Rep, Oct 11;20*(12):108

Zehetmair C, Nagy E, Leetz C, et al. (2020). Self-Practice of Stabilizing and Guided Imagery Techniques for Traumatized Refugees via Digital Audio Files: Qualitative Study. *J Med Internet Res, Sep 23;22*(9):e17906

5.3   Visit 3: Rescripting

5.3.1   Rescripting Clinic Talking Points

- How did it go with practicing positive imagery?
- Let's review your nightmare logs
- Did you notice any new trends?
- Were there any new or ongoing triggers you noticed?
- Did the positive imagery change any aspects of your data?
- Today we will take the concept of imaging a scene in your mind's eye one step further
- We will review the concept of *rescripting* which is the technique we use to address nightmares

- Today we will go through the exercise, and I will take notes while walking you through the process
- By the end of our visit, there will be a typed scene to share with you which you will rehearse for homework
- Rescripting:
    - Rescripting involves taking the content from the start of your nightmare—i.e., before it *turns bad* and changing the content after that point
    - First let's select a nightmare to rescript
        Without sharing details, can you give a title to a nightmare that you have frequently? Perhaps the nightmare that is causing the most distress
    - Now we need to identify the "hot spot"—this is the point we are referring to—after this point, the dream turns into a nightmare—it can be a sound, sight, interaction, etc.
        For example, a veteran shared that his dream starts off with him and his buddy walking on a path in Iraq, talking about their hometowns and families—when suddenly, he *hears a loud noise...*
        In this example the *loud noise* is this veteran's hot spot
        What is your hotspot?
    - Next, we need to detail all content, in full vivid detail, that occurs before the hot spot
        For the veteran example, he shared all details of what occurred before the loud sound
        From your experience, can you share all details you can think of that occurred before your hotspot?
        - What did you see? Who was there? What was around you? How was the temperature? Any smells? What did you hear? What kind of interactions occurred?
    - The final step is to invent a different ending—and go through all such details
        Back to the veteran example, he decided that when he heard the loud noise, he looked ahead, and all of his friends and family were at a huge barbeque with fireworks and it was the 4th of July
        Use your imagination and let's come up with a brand-new ending after your hotspot
        - What happens next? Who is there? What do you see? What is there? Any smells? How is the temperature? How do you feel? What kind of interactions occur?
- Now that we have a detailed rescript typed up, I will share this with you and you can practice this from home
- We want you to do 10-15-minute practice sessions 2 times per day
- Some people choose to do this right before going to sleep while others prefer to only do practice sessions during the day
- If you find that your rescript evokes any negative emotions, make modifications accordingly
- You might think of people or items that help you feel safe and secure to add as details to your rescript

- In addition, twice per day practices of rescripting, we also want you to continue to complete nightmare logs each morning

5.3.2   Rescripting Reading List

Davis JL, Rhudy JL, Pruiksma KE, et al. (2011). Physiological predictors of response to exposure, relaxation, and rescripting therapy for chronic nightmares in a randomized clinical trial. *J Clin Sleep Med. Dec 15;7*(6):622–31.

Long ME, Davis JL, Springer JR, et al. (2011). The role of cognitions in imagery rescripting for posttraumatic nightmares. *J Clin Psychol. Oct;67*(10):1008–16.

Pruiksma KE, Cranston CC, Rhudy JL, et al. (2018). Randomized controlled trial to dismantle exposure, relaxation, and rescripting therapy (ERRT) for trauma-related nightmares. *Psychol Trauma, Jan;10*(1):67–75.

Waltman SH, Shearer D, & Moore BA (2018). Management of Post-Traumatic Nightmares: a Review of Pharmacologic and Nonpharmacologic Treatments Since 2013. *Curr Psychiatry Rep, Oct 11;20*(12):108.

Kunze AE, Arntz A, Morina N, et al. (2017). Efficacy of imagery rescripting and imaginal exposure for nightmares: A randomized wait-list controlled trial. *Behav Res Ther, Oct;97*:14–25.

Kunze AE, Lancee J, Morina N, et al. (2016). A. Efficacy and mechanisms of imagery rescripting and imaginal exposure for nightmares: study protocol for a randomized controlled trial. *Trials, Sep 26;17*(1):469.

Kunze AE, Lancee J, Morina N, et al. (2019). Mediators of Change in Imagery Rescripting and Imaginal Exposure for Nightmares: Evidence From a Randomized Wait-List Controlled Trial. *Behav Ther, Sep;50*(5):978–993.

5.4   Visit 4: Rescripting Follow-up

5.4.1   Rescripting Follow-up Clinic Talking Points

- How did it go with practicing rescripting?
- Let's review your nightmare logs
- Did you notice any new trends?
- Were there any new or ongoing triggers you noticed?
- Did the rescripting change any aspects of your data?
- Today we will go through the original nightmare rescript and see if there is any need for adjustments
  - Did any of your rescripting sessions evoke negative emotions?
  - What changes can we make to the rescript so that negative emotions are not evoked?
  - Ideally, the rescript is either a neutral experience or evokes positive emotions
- Now that you have an adjusted rescript, please practice this version twice per day between now and our next visit

- If it has been 2 weeks and the original nightmare has not occurred, or has significantly reduced in severity, you can move to rescripting a different nightmare
- Remember to continue keeping nightmare logs

5.5 Visit 5: Maintenance and Relapse Prevention

5.5.1 Maintenance and Relapse Prevention Clinic Talking Points

- How did it go with practicing rescripting?
- Let's review your nightmare logs
- Did the rescripting change any aspects of your data?
- Today is our final session
- We have gone through the core components of Imagery Rehearsal Therapy
- Reminders for maintaining gains:
  - Let's review the key components of our nightmare education handout—any remaining questions?
  - How are you doing with sleep habits and general sleep hygiene? Any additional goals you might have?
  - We want you to continue to use the positive imagery technique as a coping technique for distress and support for any remaining insomnia
  - As discussed in our last visit, we want you to continue to practice rescripting twice per day until the original nightmare is no longer occurring, or is significantly less distressing
  - Continue adjusting the rescript if any negative emotions are evoked
  - Add supportive people or objects that feel calming or empowering
  - If it has been 2 weeks and you have not had the original nightmare, or it is significantly less distressing, you can then move to rescript another nightmare
- Troubleshooting ongoing symptoms:
  - For most patients, the rescript infiltrates, or takes the place of the original nightmare after consistent practice
  - If you are not experiencing any relief from use of rescripting, consider the following:
      Work with a psychologist on potential ongoing PTSD symptoms
      Inquire with a prescribing physician about whether medication adjustments (e.g., medications that might impact REM sleep) or Prazosin (i.e., which may support nightmare reduction) could be appropriate
      Consider whether any underlying mood or medical symptoms need further attention
- Preventing relapse:
  - If you are experiencing relief, remember that there is risk of nightmare relapse
  - Nightmare relapse can occur when triggers are not adequately managed
  - In the past several weeks, what have you noted as your most common triggers?
  - What steps can be taken to minimize the impact of such triggers or cope with triggers when they occur?

- Treatment wrap-up:
  - Do you have any questions leftover?
  - Please feel free to return for booster sessions as needed if relapse of symptoms occurs

Bibliography

1. American Academy of Sleep Medicine. International classification of sleep disorders 3rd ed (2014). Darien, IL American Academy of Sleep Medicine, 257.

Delayed Sleep Phase Syndrome

6

6.1 Provider Guide to Assessment

Given that the most common circadian rhythm disorder seen by Behavioral Sleep Medicine Specialists is Delayed Sleep Phase Syndrome (DSPS), we will focus on that disorder.

Assessment:
- Often patients who you end up diagnosing with DSPS were initially referred or presenting with insomnia or excessive daytime sleepiness
- During an intake with such patients, you may suspect DSPS for the following reasons:
    - Your patient struggles with falling asleep but denies prolonged awakenings
    - On weekends and vacations, when patient can go to bed later, they fall asleep faster
- For some patients, you can confirm a diagnosis through the intake process whereas you might need to first collect data for confirmation for others (e.g., actigraphy, sleep logs)
    - The Morningness-Eveningness Questionnaire is a commonly used tool to support confirmation of DSPS
- Many patients will have DSPS, insomnia and poor sleep hygiene
- It is important to clarify whether comorbid behavioral sleep medicine symptoms are present as this will impact your treatment plan

The Figures 6.1, 6.2, and 6.3, patient handouts, clinic talking points, and diagnostic criteria are shown below to help with the understanding and working with Delayed Sleep Phase Syndrome.

6.2   Delayed Sleep-Wake Phase Disorder Diagnostic Criteria

6.2.1   Delayed Sleep-Wake Phase Disorder

ICD-9-CM code: 327.31   ICD-10-CM code: G47.21

Diagnostic Criteria
Criteria A–E must be met

A. There is a significant delay in the phase of the major sleep episode in rela-
   tion to the desired or required sleep time and wake-up time, as evidenced
   by a chronic or recurrent complaint by the patient or a caregiver of inabil-
   ity to fall asleep and difficulty awakening at a desired or required
   clock time.
B. The symptoms are present for at least 3 months.
C. When patients are allowed to choose their ad libitum schedule, they will
   exhibit improved sleep quality and duration for age and maintain a delayed
   phase of the 24-h sleep-wake pattern.
D. Sleep log Possible, after graphy monitoring for at least 7 Days (preferably
   14 days from to seize demonstrate a delay in the timing of the habitual
   sleep period. Both work/school days and free days must be included
   within this monitoring.
E. The sleep disturbance is not better explained by another current sleep disorder, medical or neurological disorder, mental disorder, medication use,
   or substance use disorder.

6.3   Circadian Rhythm Screening Tool

Morningness-Eveningness Questionnaire

Instructions:
1. Please read each question very carefully before answering.
2. Answer ALL questions.
3. Answer questions in numerical order.
4. Each question should be answered independently of others. Do NOT go back and check your answers.
5. All questions have a selection of answers. For each question, place a cross alongside ONE answer only. Some questions have a scale instead of a selection of answers. Place a cross at the appropriate point along the scale.
6. Please answer each question as honestly as possible. Both your answers and the results will be kept, in strict confidence.
7. Please feel free to make any comments in the section provided below each question.

The Questionnaire with scores for each choice

1. Considering only your own "feeling best" rhythm, at what time would you get up if you were entirely free to plan your day?

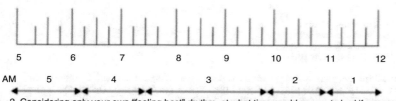

2. Considering only your own "feeling best" rhythm, at what time would you go to bed if you were entirely free to plan your evening?

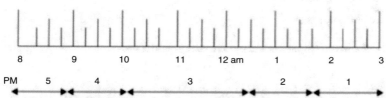

3. If there is a specific time at which you have to get up in the morning, to what extent are you dependent on being woken up by an alarm clock?

- 4   Not at all dependent
- 3   Slightly dependent
- 2   Fairly dependent
- 1   Very dependent

4. Assuming adequate environmental conditions, how easy do you find getting up in the morning?

- 1   Not at all easy
- 2   Not very easy
- 3   Fairly easy
- 4   Very easy

Fig. 6.1 This assessment tool is used to assess the extent to which a patient is more delayed or advanced with regards to their sleep phase

5. How alert do you feel during the first half hour after having woken in the morning?

- 1   Not at all alert
- 2   Slightly alert
- 3   Fairly alert
- 4   Very alert

6. How is your appetite during the first half hour after having woken up in the morning?

- 1   Very poor
- 2   Fairly poor
- 3   Fairly good
- 4   Very good

7. During the first half hour after having woken in the morning, how tired do you feel?

- 1   Very tired
- 2   Fairly tired
- 3   Fairly refreshed
- 4   Very refreshed

8. When you have no commitments the next day, at what time do you go to bed compared to your usual bedtime?

- 4   Seldom or never later
- 3   Less than one hour later
- 2   1-2 hours later
- 1   More than two hours later

9. you have decided to engage in some physical exercise. A friend suggests that you do this one hour twice a week and the best time for him is between 7:00-8:00 a.m. Bearing in mind nothing else but your own "feeling better" rhythm, how do you think you would perform?

- 4   Would be on good form
- 3   Would be on reasonable form
- 2   Would find it difficult
- 1   Would find it very difficult

10. At what time in the evening do you feel tired and as a result in need of sleep?

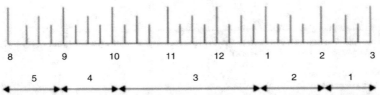

11. You wish to be at your peak performance for a test which you know is going to be mentally exhausting and lasts for two hours. You are entirely free to plan your day and considering only your own "feeling best" rhythm, which ONE of the four testing times would you choose?

- 6   8:00-10:00 a.m.
- 4   11:00 a.m.-1:00 p.m.
- 2   3:00-5:00 p.m.
- 0   7:00-9:00 p.m.

Fig. 6.1   (continued)

12. If you went to bed at 11 p.m. at what level of tiredness would you be?

- 0   Not at all tired
- 2   A little tired
- 3   Fairly tired
- 5   Very tired

13. For some reason you have gone to bed several hours later than usual, but there is no need to get up at any particular time the next morning. Which one of the following events are you most likely to experience?

- 4   Will wake up at usual time and will NOT fall asleep
- 3   Will wake up at usual time and will doze thereafter
- 2   Will wake up at usual time but will fall asleep again
- 1   Will NOT wake up until later than usual

14. One night you have to remain awake between 4-6 a.m. in order to carry out a night watch. You have no commitments the next day. Which ONE of the following alternatives will suit you best?

- 1   Would not go to bed until watch was over
- 2   Would take a na before and sleep after
- 3   Would take a good sleep before and nap after
- 4   Would take ALL sleep before watch

15. You have to do two hours of hard physical work. You are entirely free to plan your day and considering only your own "feeling best" rhythm, which ONE of the following times would you choose?

- 4   8:00-10:00 a.m.
- 3   11:00 a.m.-1:00 p.m.
- 2   3:00-5:00 p.m.
- 1   7:00-9:00 p.m.

16. You have decided to engage in hard physical exercise. A friend suggests that you do this for one hour twice a week and the best time for him is between 10-11 p.m. Bearing in mind nothing else but your own "feeling best" rhythm, how well do you think you would perform?

- 1   Would be on good form
- 2   Would be on reasonable form
- 3   Would find it difficult
- 4   Would find it very difficult

17. Suppose that you can choose your own work hours. Assume that you work a FIVE hour day (including breaks) and that your job was interesting and paid by results. Which FIVE CONSECUTIVE HOURS would you select?

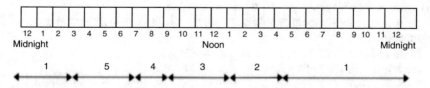

Fig. 6.1 (continued)

18. At what time of the day do you think that you reach your "feeling best" peak?

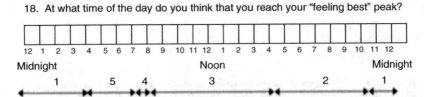

19. One hears about "morning" and "evening" types of people. Which ONE of these types do you consider yourself to be?

- 6   Definitely a "morning" type
- 4   Rather more a "morning" than an "evening" type
- 2   Rather more an "evening" than a "morning" type
- 0   Definitely an "evening" type

Fig. 6.1 (continued)

6.4   Delayed Sleep Phase Syndrome Clinic Talking Points

- Let's first discuss what it means to have a delayed sleep phase syndrome (DSPS) diagnosis

Psychoeducation:
- DSPS means that your body's internal clock, or circadian rhythm, is out of sync with what school, work or society is requiring
- Patients like you have more than a 2-h difference in when you feel sleepy, compared to when you need to sleep (e.g., you feel sleepy at 1:00 AM but you need to go to sleep by 11:00 PM to get enough sleep for your age group)
- This might also mean that there is at least a 2-h difference in when you need to wake up, compared to when you feel alert (e.g., you wake at 7:00 AM but feel excessively sleepy until 9:00 AM)
- Melatonin is the hormone produced by the suprachiasmatic nucleus which tells the brain when to feel sleepy and when to feel alert
- Cues from our environment or habits can trigger the brain to start or stop producing melatonin
  - Light tells the brain to stop producing Melatonin
  - Darkness tells the brain to start producing Melatonin
  - Social engagement, meals and activity tell the brain to stop producing Melatonin
  - Time to yourself and sedentary activities tell the brain to start producing Melatonin
- Consequences of DSPS include
  - Sleep loss resulting in mood symptoms, cognitive symptoms, low energy, and health consequences
  - Insomnia and related distress

- Late for work or school
- Decreased work or school performance in the morning

Lifestyle Changes: *Instead of treating DSPS, why not accommodate your body clock?*
- Before we dive into how to treat your DSPS, we first need to consider *whether to* treat your DSPS
- Given the challenges of maintaining treatment gains with DSPS, you may consider shifting your lifestyle to accommodate your body clock
- While we can review evidence-based treatment to advance your sleep phase and help you fall asleep and wake earlier, if you stay up late on a weekend night, you will be "back to square one"
- Here are some examples of ways that patients have instead elected to instead, accommodate their body clock
  - Submit documentation to school and request delayed start
  - Rally parents to advocate for later school start times for teens
  - Submit documentation to employer and request delayed start
  - Consider career options that can accommodate a late start and end to the workday
  - Request family support for morning responsibilities (e.g., spouse takes children to school, and you take care of bedtimes)

Sleep Hygiene
- If you have considered all options for accommodating your body clock and still decided to treat your DSPS, you will have a couple options for shifting your sleep phase
- Before we review those options and interventions, we first must make sure that your sleep hygiene is optimized
- Let's review the sleep hygiene worksheet and problem-solve any barriers to adherence

Chronotherapy
- Once you are adherent with sleep hygiene changes, next you need to select a method to shift your sleep phase - chronotherapy is one method to choose from
- To try chronotherapy, you will need to delay bedtime and waketime by 3 hours every night until you arrive at your desired bedtime
- For example, if you naturally fall asleep at 3:00 AM and wake at 11:00 AM, but your desired schedule is 10:00 PM – 6:00 AM, you would be assigned the following:
  - Day 1: 6:00 AM—2:00 PM
  - Day 2: 9:00 AM—5:00 PM
  - Day 3: 12:00 PM—8:00 PM
  - Day 4: 3:00 PM—11:00 PM
  - Day 5: 6:00 PM—2:00 AM
  - Day 6: 9:00 PM—5:00 AM
  - Day 7: 10:00 PM—6:00 AM

- If you are in school or working, this typically requires some days off
- Some patients who report staying up all night have been able to go through the process faster as they do not need to gradually work up to staying awake until the next day
- If you have any peers that struggle with the same issue, you may choose to complete the protocol at the same time as the support will help with adherence

Gradual Phase Advancement
- If taking days off is not feasible, another option is use gradual phase advancement
- This method is like chronotherapy, but involves working around the clock in the opposite direction
- Every 1–3 days, shift bedtime and waketime 15–60 minutes earlier, until you arrive at the desired sleep schedule
- Let's discuss what is realistic and feasible for you, given your schedule and current motivation to stick with the plan

Naps
- While you go through your phase shifting treatment, you must make sure to avoid all naps
- Unfortunately, taking even a short nap will deter your progress significantly
- As soon as you notice your head is feeling heavy, eyes are starting to close or you are starting to yawn, stand up and walk around
- Let's brainstorm ways to support nap avoidance…

Light therapy
- While going through a gradual phase advancement protocol, you may also benefit from morning light therapy
- Some studies suggest blue spectrum light at ~5000–10,000 lux is most effective for circadian entrainment
- It is often recommended to use light therapy immediately upon waking for 15–30 minutes
- We do not want you looking directly into the light box, but instead have it at a 30-degree angle, at arm's length distance
- Patients with a history of manic episodes, seizures or migraines should be cautious about considering light therapy

Melatonin
- Alongside your phase advancement plan, you can also try use of Melatonin to support phase entrainment
- We suggest taking a small dose (e.g., 0.5 mg – 1 mg) 4–5 hours before your natural peak in sleepiness
- For example, if you naturally feel sleepy at 2:00 AM, you could take Melatonin at 9:00 PM
- Taking a higher dose risks you experiencing sleepiness earlier than planned
- In theory, as you shift your sleep schedule, you also shift the time you take Melatonin because we are assuming that your circadian rhythm is aligning with the schedule shifting efforts

Cognitive Behavioral Treatment for Insomnia
- We want you to keep track of your sleep using sleep logs while implementing the changes discussed
- At our follow-up visit, we will review your sleep log data, and typically provide 2–3 sessions for support and customization
- If insomnia is revealed at follow-up, despite phase shifting adherence, we would then proceed with the 5–8 sessions from the CBT-I protocol [see earlier chapter]

6.5   Delayed Sleep Phase Syndrome Sleep Hygiene Handout

This is a handout Dr. Medalie sends home with patients at the culmination of their initial behavioral consultation.

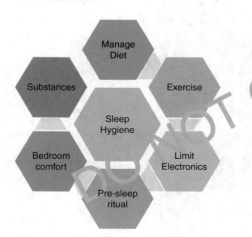

Diet: Avoid heavy meals within 3 hours of bedtime

Exercise: Regular exercise supports optimal sleep - minimize exercise within 3 hours of bedtime

Electronics: Turn off devices 1 hour before bedtime - leave them off

Pre-sleep ritual: Hot bath/shower, soft music, light reading before bedtime

Bedroom comfort: White noise machine, cool temperature, black-out shades

Substances: Minimize "night caps", limit nicotine before bedtime/during sleep window, stop caffeine 6-10 hours before bedtime

6.6   Delayed Sleep Phase Syndrome Tracking

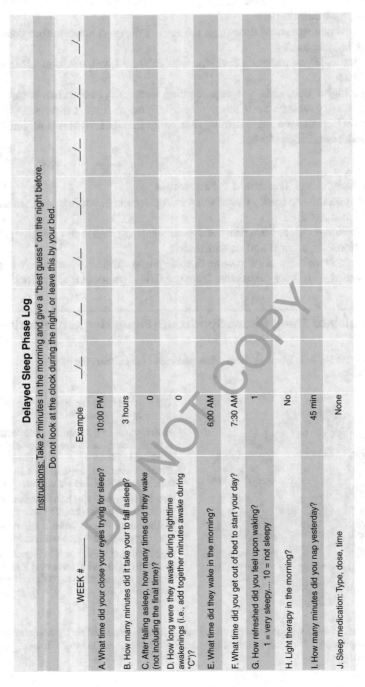

Delayed Sleep Phase Log

Instructions: Take 2 minutes in the morning and give a "best guess" on the night before. Do not look at the clock during the night, or leave this by your bed.

WEEK # _____	Example						
A. What time did your close your eyes trying for sleep?	10:00 PM	_/_	_/_	_/_	_/_	_/_	_/_
B. How many minutes did it take your to fall asleep?	3 hours						
C. After falling asleep, how many times did they wake (not including the final time)?	0						
D. How long were they awake during nighttime awakenings (i.e., add together minutes awake during "C")?	0						
E. What time did they wake in the morning?	6:00 AM						
F. What time did you get out of bed to start your day?	7:30 AM						
G. How refreshed did you feel upon waking? 1 = very sleepy.... 10 = not sleepy	1						
H. Light therapy in the morning?	No						
I. How many minutes did you nap yesterday?	45 min						
J. Sleep medication: Type, dose, time	None						

Fig. 6.2 This sleep log is used by patients tracking their perceived sleep during their work addressing their delayed sleep phase symptoms. Printing and use of this handout is not permitted unless directly approved by Dr. Medalie. If interested in accumulating BSM hours or referring patients, Dr. Medalie might be able to help—https://drlullaby.com/

6.7 Delayed Sleep Phase Syndrome Patient Handout

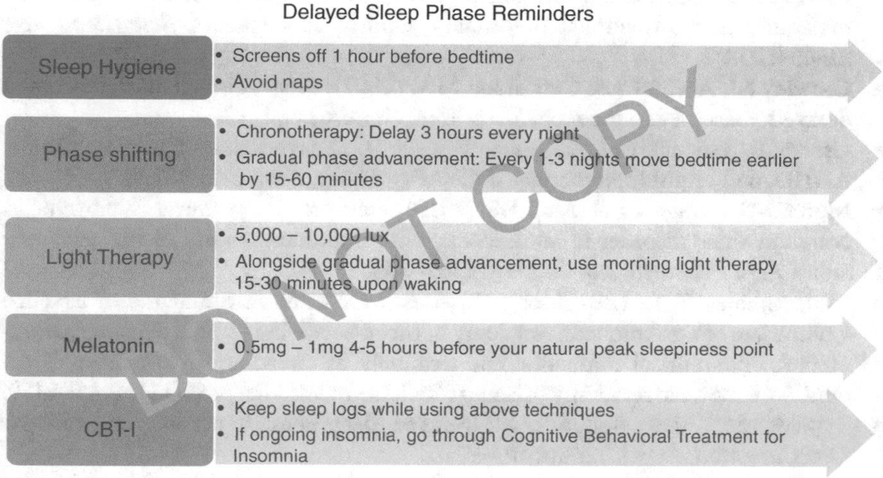

Delayed Sleep Phase Reminders

Sleep Hygiene	• Screens off 1 hour before bedtime • Avoid naps
Phase shifting	• Chronotherapy: Delay 3 hours every night • Gradual phase advancement: Every 1-3 nights move bedtime earlier by 15-60 minutes
Light Therapy	• 5,000 – 10,000 lux • Alongside gradual phase advancement, use morning light therapy 15-30 minutes upon waking
Melatonin	• 0.5mg – 1mg 4-5 hours before your natural peak sleepiness point
CBT-I	• Keep sleep logs while using above techniques • If ongoing insomnia, go through Cognitive Behavioral Treatment for Insomnia

Fig. 6.3 This handout is sent home with patients as reminders for what behavioral strategies are evidence-based in the management of delayed sleep phase syndrome. Printing and use of this handout is not permitted unless directly approved by Dr. Medalie. If interested in accumulating BSM hours or referring patients, Dr. Medalie might be able to help—https://drlullaby.com/

## 6.8	Delayed Sleep Phase Syndrome Reading List

- Auld F, Maschauer EL, Morrison I, et al. (2017). Evidence for the efficacy of melatonin in the treatment of primary adult sleep disorders. *Sleep Med Rev, Aug*;34:10–22.
- Crowley SJ, Acebo C, & Carskadon MA. (2007). Sleep, circadian rhythms, and delayed phase in adolescence. *Sleep Med, Sep;8*(6):602–12.
- Gruber R, Grizenko N, & Joober R. (2007). Delayed sleep phase syndrome, ADHD, and bright light therapy. *J Clin Psychiatry, Feb;68*(2):337–8.
- Moreno-Galarraga L, & Katz ES (2019). Delayed Sleep Phase Syndrome: A common sleep disorder in adolescents, with important quality of life repercussions. *Aten Primaria, Jun-Jul;51*(6):387–388.
- Morgenthaler, T. I., Lee-Chiong, T., Alessi, C., et al. & Standards of Practice Committee of the American Academy of Sleep Medicine (2007). Practice parameters for the clinical evaluation and treatment of circadian rhythm sleep disorders. An American Academy of Sleep Medicine report. *Sleep*, *30*(11), 1445–1459.
- Typaldos M, (2019). Sockrider M. Delayed Sleep Phase Syndrome. *Am J Respir Crit Care Med. Aug 15;200*(4):P7-P8.
- van Maanen A, Meijer AM, van der Heijden KB, et al. (2016). The effects of light therapy on sleep problems: A systematic review and meta-analysis. *Sleep Med Rev, Oct*;29:52–62.
- Wyatt JK (2004). Delayed sleep phase syndrome: pathophysiology and treatment options. *Sleep, Sep 15*;27(6):1195–203.

Bibliography

1. American Academy of Sleep Medicine. International Classification of Sleep Disorders. 3rd ed. Darien, IL: American Academy of Sleep Medicine; 2014. p. 191.
2. Horne JA, Östberg O. A self-assessment questionnaire to determine morningness-eveningness in human circadian rhythms. Int J Chronobiol. 1976;4:97–110.

Night Eating Syndrome

7

7.1 Night Eating Syndrome Clinic Talking Points

- Given that you shared you need to eat a snack to return to sleep, and that this is causing distress, it sounds like you have features of Night Eating Syndrome (NES)
- We can start off your treatment with some important teaching points about this problem

Psychoeducation
- NES accompanies sleep maintenance insomnia when patients feel they can not return to sleep unless they eat
- With this repeated relationship between eating and return to sleep, nighttime awakenings become further associated with this intense urge for consuming calories
- Furthermore, when patients consider the option of not eating, they fear insomnia, and this fear of insomnia can then turn into a self-fulfilling prophecy (i.e., not eating makes it harder to return to sleep) because of that fear response
- With the increase in calories consumed during the night, patients then waking feeling full
- They often then do not feel hungry for breakfast or lunch
- With less calories consumed during the day, the desire for more calories at night increases, making them more vulnerable to repeated night eating
- This problem can lead to weight gain, anxiety, and insomnia
- Before we proceed with learning interventions, let's first make sure we are not missing a diagnosis that might be more appropriate:
    - *Sleep Eating*: When you have events involving calorie consumption at night, do you remember these events the next day?

L. Medalie, *Behavioral Sleep Medicine*,
https://doi.org/10.1007/978-3-031-12574-4_7

If not, you might instead have a parasomnia referred to as *Sleep Eating*. Patients taking sleep medications can sometimes be more at risk for such symptoms. You may benefit from talking with a sleep MD, or your prescribing physician (if you are taking a prescription sleep medication) about this issue

- *Binge eating*: Do you find yourself ingesting large quantities of food during night eating? Are you struggling to stop eating during such events, and eating after feeling full? Are these events happening during the day and night?

  If so, you might instead have a Binge Eating Disorder and may benefit from seeing an eating disorders specialist or health psychologist to address such symptoms

- *Bulimia*: After eating, do you vomit, use laxatives or exercising excessively?

  If so, you might instead have *Bulimia,* and may benefit from seeing an eating disorders specialist to address such symptoms

Cognitive Behavioral Treatment for Insomnia (CBT-I), Customized to NES
- Before we initiate the standard CBT-I protocol, let's review some ways that our approach will be modified and customized
- Throughout our 5-8 sessions, I will remind you of these customizations and integrate them into our work

Diet
- The first tip for stopping the NES cycle is to increase daytime calories
- If you consume sufficient daytime calories, your nighttime cravings for calories will decrease
- Initially, you will need to eat breakfast and lunch without a high appetite to start the cycle, but eventually, your appetite peaks will return to standard timings
- What is your goal for timed breakfast, lunch and dinner?
- Please set a cell phone alarm reminder for your mealtimes to help keep you on track
- Some patients benefit from working with a dietician alongside such changes

Thoughts, Emotions, Behaviors
- *Example:* The thought **"I must eat to return to sleep"** triggers the emotion ***anxiety,*** which results in the behavior **snacking** then returning to sleep.
- To break the cycle, you will learn to challenge the thought (e.g., cognitive restructuring), de-escalate the emotion (e.g., relaxation strategies) and replace the behavior (e.g., stimulus control)

Medication
- Depending on how things go, some patients struggling to break the NES cycle benefit from taking an SSRI medication
- Please talk to your prescribing physician or consider talking with a psychiatrist about whether this might be helpful

Tracking
- Throughout our work together, we will have you track sleep and food intake
- Making sure you keep up with regular breakfast, lunch and dinner will support our progress with treatment

The figures 7.1, 7.2, 7.3 and 7.4, patient handouts, clinic talking points, and diagnostic criteria are shown below to help with the understanding and working with Night Eating Syndrome.

7.2   Proposed Diagnostic Criteria for Night Eating Syndrome

A. The daily pattern of eating demonstrated a significantly increased intake in the evening and/pr nighttime, a manifested by one or both of the following:
   1. at least 25% of food intake is consumed after the evening meal.
   2. At least two episodes of nocturnal eating per week.
B. Awareness and recall of evening and nocturnal eating episodes are present.
C. The clinical picture is characterized by at least three of the following features:
   1. Lack of desire to eat in the morning and/or breakfast is omitted on four or more mornings per week.
   2. Presence of a strong urge to eat between dinner and sleep onset and/or during the night
   3. Sleep onset and/or sleep maintenance insomnia are present four or more nights per week.
   4. Presence of a belief that one must eat inorder to initiate or return to sleep.
   5. Mood is frequently depressed and/or mood worsens in the evening.
D. The disorder is associated with significant distress and/or impairment in functioning.
E. The disordered pattern of eating had been maintained for at least 3 months.
F. The disorder is not secondary to substance abuse or dependence, medical disorder, medication, or another psychiatric disorder.
   1. at least 25% of food intake is consumed after the evening meal.
   2. At least two episodes of nocturnal eating per week.

Fig. 7.1 This is a questionnaire used during CBT for Night Eating Syndrome treatment. It can be used to measure the degree of symptoms present

7.3   Night Eating Questionnaire

Night Eating Questionnaire
Directions: Please circle ONE answer for each question.

1. How hungry are you usually in the morning?

0	1	2	3	4
Not at all	A little	Somewhat	Moderately	Very

2. When do you usually eat for the final time?

0	1	2	3	4
Before 9 am	9:01 to 12 pm	12:01 to 3 pm	3:01 to 6 pm	6:01 or later

3. Do you have cravings or urges to eat snacks after supper, but before bedtime?

0	1	2	3	4
Not at all	A little	Somewhat	Very much so	Extremely so

4. How much control do you have over your eating between supper and bedtime?

0	1	2	3	4
None at all	A little	Some	Very much	Complete

5. How much of your daily food intake do you consume *after* suppertime?

0	1	2	3	4
0%	1-25%	26-50%	51-75%	76-100%
(none)	(up to a quarter)	(about half)	(more than half)	(almost all)

6. Are you currently feeling blue or down in the dumps?

0	1	2	3	4
Not at all	A little	Somewhat	Very much so	Extremely

7. When you are feeling blue, is your mood lower in the: _____ check if your mood does not change during the day

0	1	2	3	4
Early morning	Late morning	Afternoon	Early evening	Late evening/nighttime

8. How often do you have trouble getting to sleep?

0	1	2	3	4
Never	Sometimes	About half the time	Usually	Always

9. Other than to use the bathroom, how many times per week will you wake at least once during the night?

0	1	2	3	4
Never	less than once a week	About once a week	More than once a week	Every night

********************** IF 0 on #9, PLEASE STOP HERE ************************

Fig. 7.2 This questionnaire is used during the CBT for Night Eating Syndrome treatment journey to measure the degree of symptoms present

10. Do you have cravings or urges to eat snacks when you wake up at night?

0	1	2	3	4
Not at all	A little	Somewhat	Very much so	Extremely so

11. Do you need to eat in order to get back to sleep when you awake at night?

0	1	2	3	4
Not at all	A little	Somewhat	Very much so	Extremely so

12. When you get up in the middle of the night, how often do you snack?

0	1	2	3	4
Never	Sometimes	About half the time	Usually	Always

*********************** IF 0 on #12, PLEASE STOP HERE ************************

13. When you snack in the middle of the night, how aware are you of your eating?

0	1	2	3	4
Not at all	A little	Somewhat	Very much so	Completely

14. How much control do you have over your eating while you are up at night?

0	1	2	3	4
Not at all	A little	Somewhat	Very much so	Complete

How long have your current difficulties with night eating been going one?
_____ mos._____years

Fig. 7.2 (continued)

7.4   Night Eating Syndrome Tracking

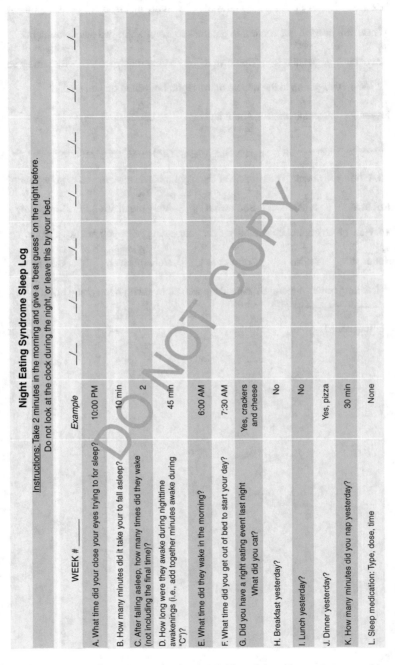

Night Eating Syndrome Sleep Log

Instructions: Take 2 minutes in the morning and give a "best guess" on the night before.
Do not look at the clock during the night, or leave this by your bed.

WEEK #	Example	_/_	_/_	_/_	_/_	_/_	_/_	_/_	_/_
A. What time did your close your eyes trying to for sleep?	10:00 PM								
B. How many minutes did it take your to fall asleep?	10 min								
C. After falling asleep, how many times did they wake (not including the final time)?	2								
D. How long were they awake during nighttime awakenings (i.e., add together minutes awake during "C")?	45 min								
E. What time did they wake in the morning?	6:00 AM								
F. What time did you get out of bed to start your day?	7:30 AM								
G. Did you have a right eating event last night What did you eat?	Yes, crackers and cheese								
H. Breakfast yesterday?	No								
I. Lunch yesterday?	No								
J. Dinner yesterday?	Yes, pizza								
K. How many minutes did you nap yesterday?	30 min								
L. Sleep medication: Type, dose, time	None								

Fig. 7.3 This log is used to track reports of eating habits, night eating symptoms and insomnia symptoms throughout the CBT for NES treatment process. Printing and use of this handout is not permitted unless directly approved by Dr. Medalie. If interested in accumulating BSM hours or referring patients, Dr. Medalie might be able to help—https://drlullaby.com/

7.5   **Night Eating Syndrome Patient Handout**

Night Eating Syndrome

Meals

After night eating, your appetite drops and you may naturally consume less calories during the day which leaves you more hungry at night. This cycle perpetuates night eating tendances

Break the cycle: consistent breakfast, lunch and dinner

Thoughts, Emotions, Behaviors

Example: The thought **"I must eat to return to sleep"** triggers the emotion *anxiety,* which results in the behavior **snacking** then returning to sleep. To break the cycle – learn to challenge the thought, de-escalate the emotion and replace the behavior choice through Cognitive Behavioral Treatment

Insomnia

Learning tools to address insomnia symptoms decreases the need for coping with the awakenings with snacks

Fig. 7.4 Dr. Medalie sends patients home with this handout to remind them of the evidence-based concepts relevant to reducing NES symptoms. Printing and use of this handout is not permitted unless directly approved by Dr. Medalie. If interested in accumulating BSM hours or referring patients, Dr. Medalie might be able to help—https://drlullaby.com/

7.6   Night Eating Syndrome Reading List

- Allison KC, & Tarves EP (2011). Treatment of night eating syndrome. *Psychiatr Clin North Am, Dec;34*(4):785-96.
- Gallant AR, Lundgren J, & Drapeau V (2012). The night-eating syndrome and obesity. *Obes Rev, Jun;13*(6):528-36.
- McCuen-Wurst C, Ruggieri M, & Allison KC (2018). Disordered eating and obesity: associations between binge-eating disorder, night-eating syndrome, and weight-related comorbidities. *Ann N Y Acad Sci, Jan;1411*(1):96-105.
- Riccobono G, Iannitelli A, Pompili A, et al. (2020). Night Eating Syndrome, circadian rhythms and seasonality: a study in a population of Italian university students. *Riv Psichiatr. Jan-Feb;55*(1):47-52.
- Townsend AB (2007). Night eating syndrome. *Holist Nurs Pract, Sep-Oct;21*(5):217-21; quiz 222.
- Yoshida J, Eguchi E, Nagaoka K, et al. (2018). Association of night eating habits with metabolic syndrome and its components: a longitudinal study. *BMC Public Health. Dec 11;18*(1):1366.

Bibliography

1. Allison KC, et al. Proposed diagnostic criteria for night eating syndrome. The International Journal of Eating Disorders. 2010;433:241–7.
2. Allison KC, Lundgren JD, O'Reardon JP, Martino NS, Sarwer DB, Wadden TA, Crosby RD, Engel SG, Stunkard AJ. The Night Eating Questionnaire (NEQ): Psychometric properties of a measure of severity of the Night Eating Syndrome. Eating Behaviors. 2008;9(1):62–72.

Parasomnias

8

8.1 Parasomnias Clinic Talking Points

This section reviews the Behavioral Sleep Medicine specialist role and process for supporting patients with parasomnias.

- Based on what you shared, the events described likely fall into the category of parasomnias
- The best way to address this problem is to teach you about parasomnias, rule-out symptoms of underlying causes and review triggers and habit changes to improve control over symptoms

8.1.1 Psychoeducation

- Parasomnias are behaviors which happen during sleep
- Many overlearned behaviors, such as talking, walking, eating, and urinating, can occur during sleep
- These events typically occur during the first third of the night, during a stage of sleep called slow wave sleep
- Typically, people do not recall these the events the following day
- When family members try to talk to people during events, patients often engage in nonsensical speech and are unable to keep eye contact or recognize family members
- We do not recommend waking up patients during sleepwalking or night terrors
  - Waking patients during events can produce confusion, agitation, and sometimes resulting insomnia
- Instead, we recommend re-directing patients back to bed
- If any safety concerns arise (e.g., sleepwalkers leaving the house), safety precautions are essential
- We always suggest reviewing your symptoms with your physician to thoroughly rule-out any medical causes for symptoms (e.g., seizures)

L. Medalie, *Behavioral Sleep Medicine*,
https://doi.org/10.1007/978-3-031-12574-4_8

8.1.2   Triggers

- Most patients find that when they learn to control triggers, they experience less frequent parasomnias
- Here are several trigger management strategies to consider:
  - *Sleep quantity*: Sleep deprived patients are more vulnerable to increased frequency of parasomnias. If you are not getting enough hours of sleep, the sleep debt will lead to you crashing into higher density slow wave sleep which means more parasomnias can occur. Let's review the handout on sleep need across ages and troubleshoot any barriers to getting adequate sleep…
  - *Sleep quality:* Sleep apnea, periodic limb movements, allergies and pain are examples of factors which can interfere with sleep quality. If sleep quality is poor, this can put you at increased risk for more frequent parasomnias. If you have symptoms that may interfere with sleep quality, we will review appropriate referrals.
  - *Stress*: Increased stress is another risk factor for triggering increased frequency of parasomnias. If persistent stress, anxiety, or mood symptoms are present, we can discuss appropriate referrals.
  - *Sick*: When patients are sick, they tend to have increased frequency of parasomnias. We always want patients to catch and manage symptoms early to maximize trigger management.
- In addition to keeping in mind general information about parasomnias, we will now review specific information pertaining to your symptoms

8.1.3   Sleepwalking

Safety proofing
- Since some patients can get hurt during sleepwalking episodes, we suggest taking precautions to prevent injury
- Put extra locks and alarms on windows and front doors
- Lock up knives in the kitchen
- Put up a gate in front of the stairs
- Bell on the door:
  - Either put a small window or door alarm on the bedroom door – or nail a bell on the bedroom door
  - This approach will allow you to know as soon as so you are alerted as soon as the patient leaves their bedroom

Scheduled awakenings
- Some families are successful with using scheduled awakenings to reduce the frequency of sleepwalking
- First, you need to keep sleep logs for 1-2 weeks to track what time the sleepwalking happens

- While keeping sleep logs, it is important that the patient keeps the same bedtime and waketime for the most accurate data collection
- Once you get a sense for what time the sleepwalking events happen:
  - Set your alarm for 30 minutes before the events typically occur
  - Wake up the patient gently, then have them return to sleep at those times

Medication
- If safety concerns are significant, you may need to talk to your prescribing physician about medication options for reducing sleepwalking

8.1.4 Sleep Terrors

Normalizing sleep terrors
- If underlying rule-outs are finalized, and no safety concerns are noted, we often explain to parents that sleep terrors can be normal, and most children grow out of them
- Sleep terrors are scary for parents, yet children have no recall of events the next day
- As reviewed earlier, we do not recommend waking children during sleep terrors
- Given that events are typically brief, in duration, if parents feel comfortable using a video monitor for safety, they do not necessarily need to even go into the room
- If they do go into the bedroom, they can simply direct the patient to lay back down

Scheduled awakenings
- If sleep terrors are disruptive to the sleep of others or causing parents significant distress, you can try use of scheduled awakenings to reduce the frequency of sleep terrors
- First, you need to keep sleep logs for 1-2 weeks to track what time the sleep terrors happen
- While keeping sleep logs, it is important that the patient keeps the same bedtime and waketime for the most accurate data collection
- Once you get a sense for what time sleep terrors:
  - Set your alarm for 30 minutes before the events typically occur
  - Wake up the patient gently, then have them return to sleep at those times

8.1.5 Sleep Enuresis

Normalizing sleep enuresis
- We typically do not diagnose sleep enuresis until patients are 7 years old

Even then, if symptoms are no impacting self-esteem or disturbing functioning there is not always a need to intervene

- It is important not to punish children or make them feel bad about symptoms, but instead remind them that many children are going through the same problem

Rule-outs

- Before confirming sleep enuresis, patients may benefit from outside referrals
- Here are some scenarios that warrant outside referrals:
  - Patient was dry for at least 3 months at night, and then started having accidents
    If trauma or psychological stress precipitated the return of bedwetting, referral to psychiatry is warranted
    If medical symptoms (e.g., constipation, urinary tract infection, etc.) precipitated the return of bedwetting, referral to urology is warranted
  - Patient is having both daytime and nighttime symptoms
  - Patient is having both urinary and stool accidents
  - Any concerns about maintaining urinary stream, pain or urgency should be further evaluated by urology

Behavioral changes

- Void before bedtime – make sure bladder is fully emptied
- Minimize liquid intake between dinner and bedtime
  - Only sips to quench thirst

Scheduled awakenings

- Some families are successful with using scheduled awakenings to reduce the frequency of sleep enuresis events
- First, you need to keep sleep logs for 1-2 weeks to track what time the sleep enuresis events happen
- While keeping sleep logs, it is important that the patient keeps the same bedtime and waketime for the most accurate data collection
- Once you get a sense for what time the sleep enuresis events happen:
  - Set your alarm for 30 minutes before the events typically occur
  - Wake up the patient gently, bring them immediately to the bathroom at those times

Bell and pad

- Instead of parents waking up children, there are products called *Bell and Pad* which can wake children
- The bedwettingstore.com is one site to find such products
- There are products that use both alarm sounds and vibration to maximize the chance of the child waking

- The goal is for the product to wake the patient at the first drop of fluid, and the child is then supposed to go to bathroom right away
- Eventually, the patient's brain learns to wake more readily during slow wave sleep when the bladder is full

Medication
- If ongoing symptoms are present after trying behavioral strategies, you may need to talk to your prescribing physician about medication options

The Figures 8.1 and 8.2, patient handouts, clinic talking points, and diagnostic criteria are shown below to help with the understanding and working with Parasomnias.

8.2   Sleepwalking Diagnostic Criteria

These criteria can be considered while evaluating parasomnias and considering differential diagnoses.

8.2.1   Sleepwalking

ICD-9-CM code: 307.46   ICD-10-CM code: F51.3

8.2.2   Alternate Names

Somnambulism.

Diagnostic Criteria
Criteria A and B must be met
  A. The disorder meets general criteria for NREM disorders of arousal.
  B. The arousals are associated with ambulation and other complex behaviors out of bed.

8.2.3   Sleep Terrors Diagnostic Criteria

Sleep Terrors

ICD-9-CM code: 307.46   ICD-10-CM code: F51.4

Alternate Names

Night terrors, pavor nocturnus.

Diagnostic Criteria

Criteria A–C must be met

A. The disorder meets general criteria for NREM disorders of arousal.
B. The arousals are characterized by episodes of abrupt terror, typically beginning with an alarming vocalisation such as frightening scream.
C. There is intense fear and signs of autonomic arousal, including mydriasis, tachycardia, tachypnea, and diaphoresis during an episode.

8.2.4   Sleep Enuresis Diagnostic Criteria

Sleep Enuresis

ICD-9-CM code: 788.36   ICD-10-CM code: N39.44

Diagnostic Criteria

Primary Sleep Enuresis—Criteria A–D must be met

A. The patient is older than five years.
B. The patient exhibits recurrent involuntary voiding during sleep, occurring at least twice a week.
C. The condition has been present for at least three months.
D. The patient has never been consistently dry during sleep.

Secondary Sleep Enuresis—Criteria A–D must be met

A. The patient is older than five years.
B. The patient exhibits recurrent involuntary voiding during sleep, occurring at least twice a week.
C. The condition has been present for at least three months.
D. The patient has previously been consistently dry during sleep for at least 6 months.

8.2.5   Parasomnias Sleep Need Handout

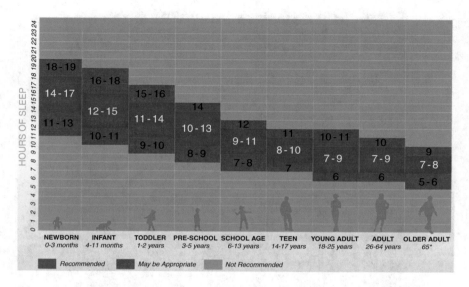

Fig. 8.1 This figure by Dr. Liela Kheirandish-Gozal's group highlights the sleep need ranges recommended by age group. As shown, there is not one set number of hours needed for specific ages, but ranges for what is recommended, and what might be appropriate. This information is extremely helpful to provide to patients, particularly knowing that adequate sleep duration can support reduced frequency and severity of parasomnias

8.2.6   Parasomnias Log

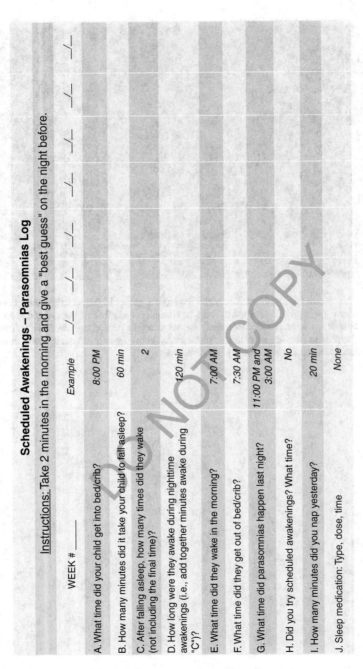

Scheduled Awakenings – Parasomnias Log

Instructions: Take 2 minutes in the morning and give a "best guess" on the night before.

WEEK # _____	Example	/	/	/	/	/	/	/
A. What time did your child get into bed/crib?	8:00 PM							
B. How many minutes did it take your child to fall asleep?	60 min							
C. After falling asleep, how many times did they wake (not including the final time)?	2							
D. How long were they awake during nighttime awakenings (i.e., add together minutes awake during "C")?	120 min							
E. What time did they wake in the morning?	7:00 AM							
F. What time did they get out of bed/crib?	7:30 AM							
G. What time did parasomnias happen last night?	11:00 PM and 3:00 AM							
H. Did you try scheduled awakenings? What time?	No							
I. How many minutes did you nap yesterday?	20 min							
J. Sleep medication: Type, dose, time	None							

Fig. 8.2 This log is an example of what Dr. Medalie sends home with patients who are struggling with parasomnias. This log allows Dr. Medalie to see if ongoing inadequate sleep duration, or other factors, might be contributing to perpetuation of parasomnias. Printing and use of this handout is not permitted unless directly approved by Dr. Medalie. If interested in accumulating BSM hours or referring patients, Dr. Medalie might be able to help—https://drlullaby.com/

8.2.7 Parasomnias Reading List

Arkin, A. M. (2018). Sleep-talking: Psychology and psychophysiology.

Byars, K. (2011). Scheduled Awakenings: A Behavioral Protocol for Treating Sleepwalking and Sleep Terrors in Children. In Perlis, M. L., Aloia, M., & Kuhn, B. R. (Eds.). *Behavioral treatments for sleep disorders: A comprehensive primer of behavioral sleep medicine interventions* (1st ed., pp.285-292). Academic Press.

Castelnovo, A., Lopez, R., Proserpio, P., et al. (2018). NREM sleep parasomnias as disorders of sleep-state dissociation. *Nature Reviews Neurology, 14*(8), 470–481.

Erickson, J., & Vaughn, B. V. (2019). Non-REM parasomnia: the promise of precision medicine. *Sleep medicine clinics, 14*(3), 363-370.

Galbiati, A., Manni, R., Terzaghi, M., et al. (2016). Disorders of arousal. *Current Sleep Medicine Reports, 2*(2), 53–63. h

Hrozanova, M., Morrison, I., & Riha, R. (2018). Adult nrem parasomnias: An update. *Clocks & Sleep, 1*(1), 87–104.

Kotagal, S. (2009). Parasomnias in childhood. *Sleep Medicine Reviews, 13*(2), 157–168.

Loddo, G., Lopez, R., Cilea, et al. (2019). Disorders of Arousal in adults: New diagnostic tools for clinical practice. *Sleep Science and Practice, 3*(1), 5.

Mindell, J. A., & Owens, J. A. (2015.). *A clinical guide to pediatric sleep: Diagnosis and management of sleep problems.* Lippincott Williams & Wilkins.

Montplaisir, J., Zadra, A., Nielsen, T., et al. (2017). *Parasomnias. In Sleep Disorders Medicine* (pp. 1087-1113). Springer, New York, NY

Singh, S., Kaur, H., Singh, S., et al. (2018). Parasomnias: A Comprehensive Review. *Cureus, 10*(12), e3807.

Bibliography

1. American Academy of Sleep Medicine. International classification of sleep disorders. 3rd ed. Darien, IL: American Academy of Sleep Medicine; 2014. p. 229.
2. American Academy of Sleep Medicine. International classification of sleep disorders. 3rd ed. Darien, IL: American Academy of Sleep Medicine; 2014. p. 230.
3. American Academy of Sleep Medicine. International classification of sleep disorders. 3rd ed. Darien, IL: American Academy of Sleep Medicine; 2014. p. 270.
4. Hirshkowitz M, Whiton K, Albert SM, Alessi C, Bruni O, Don Carlos L, Hazen N, Herman J, Katz ES, Kheirandish-Gozal L, Neubauer DN, O'Donnell AE, Ohayon M, Peever J, Rawding R, Sachdeva RC, Setters B, Vitiello MV, Ware JC, Adams Hillard PJ. National Sleep Foundation's sleep time duration recommendations: methodology and results summary. Sleep Health. 2015;1(1):40–3.

Society for Behavioral Sleep Medicine (SBSM) Resources

9

9.1 SBSM Resource List Link

As providers embark on the journey of learning and practicing Behavioral Sleep Medicine tools, reading through the pivotal research studies, literature reviews and texts is essential. Please type the following into your browser to access the Society for Behavioral Sleep Medicine's most current resource list:

https://www.behavioralsleep.org/images/pdf/2021/Bibliography-Reading ListFinal.pdf

9.2 Theories

There are several theories that Behavioral Sleep Medicine providers must understand to effectively teach and implement research-backed strategies in our field. Knowing the theories well enough to teach them to patients, is a powerful way to motivate change. For example, understanding classical conditioning and teaching about the study of Pavlov's research on the digestive processes of dogs, is helpful in teaching stimulus control during the CBT-I protocol. Refreshing on the concepts of operant conditioning, and the Skinner Box, can help with teaching parents about the importance of behavior charts. Explaining spontaneous recovery and extinction burst theories can prepare parents before implementing behavioral strategies which teach babies and toddlers independent sleep. Thorough review of these theories will also be essential for success in your board examination performance.

9.2.1   Classic and Operant Conditioning

McSweeney, F.K., & Murphy, E. S. (2014). *The Wiley Blackwell handbook of operant and classical conditioning*. John Wiley & Sons. *Chap. 14: Characteristics, Theories, and Implications of Dynamic Changes in Reinforcer Effectiveness

Meltzer, L.J., & McLaughlin Crabtree, V. (2015). *Pediatric sleep problems: A clinician's guide to behavioral interventions*. American Psychological Association.

Sherlin, L. H., Arns, M., Lubar, J., et al. (2011). Neurofeedback and basic learning theory: Implications for research and practice. *Journal of Neurotherapy, 15*(4), 292–304.

9.2.2   Shaping/Exposure

Leggett, M.K. (2016). A Brief Review of Claustrophobia and Continuous Positive Airway Pressure (CPAP) Therapy for Sleep Apnea. *Journal of Sleep Medicine Disorders, 3*(2), 1043.

Meltzer, L.J., & McLaughlin Crabtree, V. (2015). *Pediatric sleep problems: A clinician's guide to behavioral interventions*. American Psychological Association.

Sadeh, A., Tikotzky, L., & Scher, A. (2010). Parenting and infant sleep. *Sleep Medicine Reviews, 14*(2), 89–96.'

Slifer, K. J., Kruglak, D., Benore, E., et al. (2007). Behavioral training for increasing preschool children's adherence with positive airway pressure: A preliminary study. *Behavioral Sleep Medicine, 5*(2), 147–175.

9.2.3   Reinforcement Schedules, Extinction, Spontaneous Recovery

McSweeney, F.K., & Murphy, E. S. (2014). *The Wiley Blackwell handbook of operant and classical conditioning*. John Wiley & Sons. *Chap. 14: Characteristics, Theories, and Implications of Dynamic Changes in Reinforcer Effectiveness.

Meltzer, L.J., & McLaughlin Crabtree, V. (2015). *Pediatric sleep problems: A clinician's guide to behavioral interventions*. American Psychological Association.

9.2.4   Placebo Effect

Perlis, M. L., McCall, W. V., Jungquist, C. R., et al. (2005). Placebo effects in primary insomnia. *Sleep Medicine Reviews, 9*(5), 381–389.

Stewart-Williams, S., & Podd, J. (2004). The placebo effect: Dissolving the expectancy versus conditioning debate. *Psychological Bulletin, 130*(2), 324–340.

Winkler, A., & Rief, W. (2015). Effect of placebo conditions on polysomnographic parameters in primary insomnia: A meta-analysis. *Sleep, 38*(6), 925–931.

9.2.5   Theories of Behavioral Change

Michie, S. F., West, R., Campbell, R., Brown, J., & Gainforth, H. (2014). *ABC of behavior change theories*. Silverback publishing.

Ogden, J. (2012). *Health Psychology: A Textbook*. McGraw-Hill Education (UK).

Webb, T. L., Sniehotta, F. F., & Michie, S. (2010). Using theories of behaviour change to inform interventions for addictive behaviours: Theories of behaviour change and addiction. *Addiction, 105*(11), 1879–1892.

9.2.6   Relaxation

Lehrer, P. M., Woolfolk, R. L., & Sime, W. E. (2007). *Principles and Practice of Stress Management (Third Edition)*. Guilford Press.

9.2.7   Acceptance & Commitment Therapy / Mindfulness

Dalrymple, K. L., Fiorentino, L., Politi, M. C., et al. (2010). Incorporating principles from acceptance and commitment therapy into cognitive-behavioral therapy for insomnia: A case example. *Journal of Contemporary Psychotherapy, 40*(4), 209–217.

Lappalainen, P., Langrial, S., Oinas-Kukkonen, H., et al. (2019). ACT for sleep - Internet-delivered self-help ACT for subclinical and clinical insomnia: A randomized controlled trial. *Journal of Contextual Behavioral Science, 12*, 119–127.

Lundh, L.-G. (2005). The role of acceptance and mindfulness in the treatment of insomnia. *Journal of Cognitive Psychotherapy, 19*(1), 29–39.

Ong, J. C., Ulmer, C. S., & Manber, R. (2012). Improving sleep with mindfulness and acceptance: A metacognitive model of insomnia. *Behaviour Research and Therapy, 50*(11), 651–660.

9.2.8   Cognitive Restructuring

Clark, D. A. (2013). Cognitive restructuring. *The Wiley handbook of cognitive behavioral therapy*. Wiley. (ch. 2)

Wolgast, M., Lundh, L.-G., & Viborg, G. (2013). Cognitive restructuring and acceptance: An empirically grounded conceptual analysis. *Cognitive Therapy and Research, 37*(2), 340–351.

9.2.9   Behavioral Activation

Martell, C., Addis, M., & Dimidjian, S. (2004). *Finding the Action in Behavioral Activation: The Search for Empirically Supported Interventions and Mechanisms of Change*. In S. C. Hayes, V. M. Follette, & M. M. Linehan (Eds.), Mindfulness and acceptance: Expanding the cognitive-behavioral tradition (p. 152–167). Guilford Press.

9.3   Physiology

Amlaner, C.J., Lesku, J. A., & Rattenborg, N.C. (2009). *The Evolution of sleep*. In Amlaner, C. J., Phil, D., & Fuller, P.M. (Eds.). Basics of sleep guide (2 nd Ed., pp. 11–19). Westchester, IL: Sleep Research

Kryger, M., Roth, T., & Dement, W. (2017). *Principles and Practice of Sleep Medicine (6th ed.)*. Elsevier (sections 1–5).

Yu, M. & Attarian, H. (2020). *Systems Physiology During Sleep*. In Montgomery-Downs, H.(Ed.). Sleep Science (pp. 33–46). Oxford University Press.

Behavioral Sleep Medicine Board Preparation

10

10.1 Becoming Certified

10.1.1 Requirements for Certification

Clinicians who successfully meet eligibility requirements and pass an examination will have met all requirements to be granted a certification in behavioral sleep medicine by the Board of Behavioral Sleep Medicine.

Eligibility Requirements for Examination

BSM certification requires a combination of appropriate educational background, clinical experience, and a passing score on the BSM examination. The following eligibility requirements outline the credentials and training necessary to sit for the BSM examination.

(a) Graduate level (masters or doctorate) degree in a health-related field from an accredited institution of higher learning (upload copy of diploma with application).
(b) All clinical professionals must be licensed in accordance with applicable federal, state, and local laws, and must act only within the scope of their state license and in accordance with the specific state practice requirements. (upload copy of license with application).
(c) Completion of ONE of the following BSM training tracks:

1. *Standard Track:* Formal SBSM-accredited graduate or post-doctoral BSM training program (upload copy of training program completion certificate with application and signed Standard Track Attestation Form). Candidates must complete the Standard Track Attestation Form included at the end of this Handbook or in the Application and have it signed by the Program/Training Director of the SBSM-accredited behavioral sleep medicine training program attended. The

candidate must provide sufficient detail to enable BSM reviewers to thoroughly and fairly review the candidate's qualifications. The candidate must then submit the Attestation Form(s) by uploading it to the Application.
2. *Alternate Track:* Equivalent training totaling 500 hours of didactic training and clinical experience.

10.1.2 Frequently Asked Questions from the SBSM

Who Is Eligible to Apply for DBSM Certification?
In general, applicants must hold a graduate degree in a health-related field, meet either Standard or Alternate Track training requirements as outlined in the eligibility criteria, and hold a current valid license to practice in their field of specialty. Individuals with a temporary license or whose practice is restricted by board sanction are not eligible to apply.

For a period of 2 years ending July 31, 2020, individuals holding a CBSM are also eligible to apply to obtain a DBSM without taking the BSM examination provided they have completed 40 continuing education hours in behavioral sleep medicine within the past 5 years. Thereafter CBSM holders will be required to apply through either Standard or Alternative Tracks and sit for examination.

What Disciplines Are Included as Eligible to Obtain a BSM Certification?
The current BSM certification reflects an interdisciplinary vision for the field of BSM. The BSM certification eligibility criteria indicate applicants must hold a master's or doctorate degree in a health-related field who meet the educational and clinical experience necessary to demonstrate competency in Behavioral Sleep Medicine. Such fields include but are not limited to psychology, clinical social work, medicine, counseling, advanced practice nursing, education, and dentistry.

Once I Obtain BSM Certification, Will I Need to Renew it?
Yes. You will need to renew your DBSM certification every 5 years. The renewal application will involve updating your practice information, verifying you currently license to practice, and documenting that within the past 5 years you have completed a minimum of 40 continuing education (CE) hours in behavioral sleep medicine. These hours may include areas such as normal and abnormal sleep, basic sleep science, differential diagnosis of sleep conditions, diagnostic monitoring tools in sleep medicine, psychological factors affecting sleep and behavioral treatments of sleep disorders.

If you do not meet CE requirements at the time of renewal you would need to take and pass the current BSM examination in order to renew your certification.

Do I Need to Take the BSM Exam to Obtain a DBSM if I Am Already Credentialed in Sleep Medicine or Sleep Dentistry?

Yes, if you do not also hold the CBSM (administered between 2003–2014 by the AASM/ABSM). For those with a CBSM credential representing specialty BSM expertise, the BBSM is offering a time-limited CBSM Holder Application until July 31, 2020 that exempts applicants with a CBSM from taking the current BSM examination who otherwise meet DBSM eligibility requirements.

Who Can I Contact to Get my Questions Answered About the BSM Exam?

For additional information to answer your specific questions, please contact info@bsmcredential.org.

Index

Printed in the United States
by Baker & Taylor Publisher Services